SPORTS MEDICINE

PEARLS OF WISDOM

Mary E. Cataletto, M.D.
Richard B. Birrer, M.D.
Bernard A. Griesemer, M.D.

NOTE

The intent of SPORTS MEDICINE Pearls of Wisdom is to serve as a study aid to improve performance on a standardized examination. It is not intended to be a source text of the knowledge base of medicine or to serve as a reference in any way for the practice of clinical medicine. Neither Boston Medical Publishing Corporation nor the editors warrant that the information in this text is complete or accurate. The reader is encouraged to verify each answer in several references. All drug use indications and dosages must be verified by the reader before administration of any compound.

Copyright © 2002 by Boston Medical Publishing Corporation, Lincoln, NE.

Printed in U.S.A.

All rights reserved, including the right of reproduction, in whole or in part, in any form.

The editors would like to extend thanks to Terri Lair for her excellent managing and editorial support.

Art Director: Maryse Charette

This book was produced using Times and Symbols fonts and computer based graphics with Macintosh® computers

ISBN: 1-58409-061-8

DEDICATION

This book is dedicated to the athletes who enjoy exercise as sport, recreation or simply to improve cardiovascular fitness, to the professionals who care for them and to the physicians and scientists who are working to advance the science of sports medicine.

M.C., R.B., & B.G.

EDITOR

Mary E. Cataletto, M.D., FAAP
Associate Professor of Clinical Pediatrics
SUNY Health Science Center at Stonybrook
Associate Director of Pediatric Pulmonology
Winthrop University Hospital
Mineola, NY

Richard B. Birrer, M.D., FAAFP, FACSM
Professor of Family Medicine
SUNY Health Sciences Center at Brooklyn, NY

Bernard A. Griesemer, M.D.
Health Tracks Center
Springfield, MO

CONTRIBUTING AUTHORS

Luis Alejo, M.D.
Chief, Division of Physical Medicine & Rehabilitation
Winthrop University Hospital
Mineola, NY

Cora Breunner, M.D., MPH
Assistant Professor of Pediatrics
University of Washington
Division of Adolescent Medicine
Department of Pediatrics
Children's Hospital & Medical Center
Seattle, WA

Ralph Della Ratta, M.D.
Assistant Professor of Medicine
SUNY Stonybrook
Attending Physician, Dept. of Medicine
Winthrop University Hospital
Mineola, NY

Robert Garafano, Ed.D.
Assistant Clinical Professor of Applied Physiology
College of Physicians & Surgeons
Columbia University
New York, NY

Michael R. Goler, M.D., MBA
Health Tracks Center
Springfield, MO

Charleen L. Ise, M.D., FAAFP
Associate Director Bayfront Family Practice Residency program
Assistant Clinical Professor
University of South Florida
CAQ Sports Medicine
St. Petersburg, FL

David Klocke, M.D.
Consultant, Assistant Professor
Department of Emergency Services
Mayo Clinic
Rochester, MN

Leonard R. Krilov, M.D.
Chief, Pediatric Infectious Diseases
Winthrop University Hospital
Mineola, NY

Kim LeBlanc, M.D., Ph.D., FAAFP, FACSM
Director, Family Practice Residency
University Medical Center
Breaux Bridge, LA
Associate Professor of Family Medicine
Louisiana State University School of Medicine
New Orleans, LA

Sean G. Levchuck, M.D.
Director
Pediatric Cardiac Catherization Laboratory
St. Francis Hospital
Roslyn, NY

Jack Levine, M.D.
Assistant Professor of Clinical Pediatrics
Albert Einstein College of Medicine
Bronx, NY

Richard Meadows, M.D.
Hanover Family Practice
Mechanicsville, VA

Joseph Moore, M.D.
Specialty Advisor to the Navy Surgeon General for Sports Medicine
Commanding Officer
Naval Medical Clinic
Pearl Harbor, HI

Charles Peterson, M.D.
Instructor, Family and Community Medicine
Medical College of Wisconsin
Fellow, Primary Care Sports Medicine
Medical College of Wisconsin
Milwaukee, WI

Mark G. Petrizzi, M.D., FAAFP
Assistant Professor, Family Practice
Virginia Commonwealth University
School of Medicine
Richmond, VA
Hanover Family Physicians
Mechanicsville, VA

Michael J. Petrizzi, M.D., FACSM
Associate Clinical Professor
Family Practice,
Virginia Commonwealth University
College of Medicine
Richmond, VA
Residency Director of the Family Practice Program
Hanover Family Physicians
Mechanicsville, VA

Stephen G. Rice, M.D., Ph.D., M.P.H., FACSM, FAAP
Program Director
Primary Care Sports Medicine Fellowship
Director
Jersey Shore Sports Medicine Center
Department of Pediatrics
Jersey Shore Medical Center
Neptune, NJ
Clinical Associate Professor of Pediatrics
Robert Wood Johnson Medical School
University of Medicine and Dentistry of New Jersey
New Brunswick, NJ

Brent S. E. Rich, M.D., ATC
CAQ, Primary Care Sports Medicine
Team Physician
2000 United States Olympic Team
University Sports Medicine
Phoenix, AZ

Eric Small, M.D., FAAP
Asst Clinical Professor
Pediatrics, Orthopedics and Rehabilitation Medicine
Mount Sinai School of Medicine
New York, NY

Kenneth Taylor – Butler, M.D., FAAFP
Faculty Physician
Trinity Family Practice Residency
Clinical Associate Professor of Family Practice
University of Missouri / Kansas City
Kansas City, MO

Russell White, M.D.
Associate Director
Family Practice Program
Director, Sports Medicine Fellowship
Bayfront Medical Center
St. Petersburg, FL
Clinical Associate Professor
Family Medicine
University of South Florida College of Medicine
Tampa, FL

WE APPRECIATE YOUR COMMENTS!

We appreciate your opinion and encourage you to send us any suggestions
or recommendations. Please let us know if you discover any errors, or if there is any way
we can make Pearls of Wisdom more helpful to you.
We are also interested in recruiting new authors and editors.
Please call, write, fax, or e-mail. We look forward to hearing from you.

Send comments to:

Boston Medical Publishing Corporation
4780 Linden Street, Lincoln, NE, 68516

888-MBOARDS (626-2737)
402-484-6118
Fax: 402-484-6552
E-mail: bmp@emedicine.com
www.bmppearls.com

INTRODUCTION

Congratulations ! Sports Medicine *Pearls of Wisdom* will help you learn about Sports Medicine as well as prepare for the Sports Medicine Board. While intended for Sports Medicine specialists, we have learned that *Pearls* unique format is also useful for house officers and medical students rotating in Sports Medicine and studying for boards or inservice examinations in the corresponding specialties of Internal Medicine, Family Practice, Orthopedic Surgery, Pediatrics and Emergency Medicine. A few words are appropriate discussing intent, format and use.

Since *Pearls* is primarily intended as a study aid, most of the text is written in rapid fire question – answer format. This way readers receive immediate gratification. Moreover misleading or confusing " foils " are not provided. This eliminates the risk of erroneously assimilating an incorrect piece of information that makes a big impression. Questions themselves often contain a " pearl " intended to reinforce the answer. Additional comments may be attached to the answer in various forms, including mneumonics, visual imagery, repetition, and humor. Additional information not requested in the question may be included in the answer. Emphasis has been placed on distilling trivia and key facts that are easily overlooked, that are quickly forgotten, and that somehow seem to be needed on board examinations.

Many questions have answers without explanations. This enhances ease of reading and rate of learning. Explanations often occur in a later question / answer. Upon reading an answer, a reader may think, " Hmm, why is that ? " or, " Are you sure ? " If this happens to you, go check ! Truly assimilating these disparate facts into a framework of knowledge absolutely requires further reading on the surrounding concepts. Information learned in response to seeking an answer to a particular question is retained better than information that is passively observed. Take advantage of this ! Use *Pearls* with your preferred source texts handy and open.

The *Sports Medicine Pearls* is presented in topic areas important to your preparation for examinations in sports medicine. This permits you to concentrate on areas of interest or weakness. Some questions will test your recall of basic facts, while others will ask you to integrate what you've learned into clinical case studies. After completing a Pearls chapter, readers are encouraged to examine the corresponding textbook chapter entirely, for comprehensiveness. Certain topics have been repeated in a single chapter and across chapters. This was intentional. Some topics are so important to a practitioner that repetition was utilized as a learning tool.

Pearls does have limitations. We have found many conflicts between sources of information. We have tried to verify in several references the most accurate information. Some texts have internal discrepancies further confounding clarification.

Pearls risks accuracy by aggressively pruning complex concepts down to the simplest kernel; the dynamic knowledge base and clinical practice of sports medicine is not like that ! Furthermore, new research and practice occasionally deviates from that which likely represents the correct answer for test purposes. This text is designed to maximize your score on a test. Refer to your most current sources of information and mentors for direction for practice.

Pearls is designed to be used, not just read. It is an interactive text. The question – answer format is most useful as an active learning tool when used in conjunction with Sports Medicine texts The more active the learning process, the better the understanding. Use a 3 x 5 card and cover the answers; attempt all questions. A study method we recommend is oral, group study. The mechanics of this method are simple and no one ever appears stupid. One person holds *Pearls*, with the answers covered, and reads the question. Each person, including the reader, says " Check " when he or she has an answer in mind. After everyone has " checked " in, someone states his/ her answer. If this answer is correct, on to the next one; if not, another person says their answer or the answer can be read. Usually the person who " checks " in first gets the first shot at stating the answer. Try it, it's almost fun !

Pearls is also designed to be re-used several times to allow, dare we use the word, memorization. Two check boxes are provided for any scheme of keeping track of questions answered correctly or incorrectly.

We welcome your comments, suggestions and criticism. Great effort has been made to verify these questions and answers. Some answers may not be the answer you would prefer. Most often this is attributable to variance between original sources. Please make us aware of any errors you find. We hope to make continuous improvements and would greatly appreciate any input with regard to format, organization, content, presentation or about specific questions.

Study hard and good luck.

M.C., R.B., & B.G.

TABLE OF CONTENTS

TEAM PHYSICIAN, ROLE AND RESPONSIBILITIES 11

MEDICAL SCIENCE
    ANATOMY AND BIOMECHANICS 15
    GROWTH AND DEVELOPMENT 33
    EXERCISE PHYSIOLOGY 45
    PHARMACOTHERAPEUTICS 63
    ERGOGENIC AIDS 69
    NUTRITION 77

CLINICAL SPORTS MEDICINE
    PREPARTICIPATION PHYSICAL EXAMINATION 87
    CONDITIONING AND TRAINING 95
    EXERCISE BENEFITS & WRITING AN EXERCISE PRESCRIPTION 101
    EPIDEMIOLOGY OF SPORTS INJURIES 111
    EVENT ADMINISTRATION 117
    INJURY PREVENTION 121
    EMERGENCY ASSESSMENT AND TRIAGE 125
    DIAGNOSIS AND TREATMENT OF ACUTE MUSCULOSKELETAL INJURIES 133
    CHRONIC MEDICAL PROBLEMS IN THE ATHLETE 145
    MUSCULOSKELETAL REHABILITATION 159

SPECIAL CONSIDERATIONS
    YOUNG ATHLETES 165
    FEMALE ATHLETES 173
    DISABLED ATHLETES 179
    SENIOR ATHLETES 189
    INFECTIOUS CONCERNS 199
    ENVIRONMENTAL CONCERNS 205

PSYCHOSOCIAL ASPECTS OF SPORTS PARTICIPATION 211

PROCEDURES
    CARDIOPULMONARY RESUSCITATION 221
    EXERCISE TESTING 227
    CASTING AND SPLINTING 233
    JOINT ASPIRATION AND INTRAARTICULAR INJECTION 241

PROTECTIVE AND SUPPORTIVE EQUIPMENT 245

BIBLIOGRAPHY 251

TEAM PHYSICIAN, ROLE AND RESPONSIBILITIES

❏❏ **Which age group suffers the most sports/ recreational related injuries?**

5-24 years.

❏❏ **Within that group what percentage of sports related injuries occurs in 5 to 14 years of age?**

30 - 32 %.

❏❏ **What is the most frequent injury type over all age groups?**

Sprains and strains.

❏❏ **What area of the body is most frequently injured in the under 6 year old age group?**

The head.

❏❏ **What types of activities cause the severest injuries?**

Collision, contact and augmented speed sports (eg sledding, cycling, skateboarding, skiing, ATV's etc).

❏❏ **In terms of injury rates how do competitive, noncompetitive, organized and unsupervised recreational sports compare?**

Competitive sports have double the average rate of injury of noncompetitive ones and unsupervised recreational activities have significantly higher injury rates than organized sports events and games. Most athletes are injured off the playing field (e.g. Playing at home or in a sand lot; doing informal sports and recreational activities).

❏❏ **What is Title IX?**

Passed in 1972 the law forbids sex discrimination in schools receiving federal funding.

❏❏ **How does the rate of injury by gender compare in sports?**

The rates of injury are higher for females in many sports (e.g. basketball, gymnastics, dance).

❏❏ **How do injury types compare by gender?**

Females suffer more sprains and dislocations while males suffer strains, fractures and contusions.

❏❏ **Who are the primary members of the sports medicine team?**

Athlete, physician, coach and athletic trainer.

❏❏ **Who are the secondary members of the sports medicine team?**

Athlete's family, friends, teammates, clinical consultants, administrative personnel and officials.

❏❏ **What is the role of the athletic trainer?**

Available in about 35% of high schools, the trainer's role is athletic safety including prevention, first aid, evaluation and rehabilitation of injuries to athletes under his/her care.

❏❏ **What are the desirable requirements to be an athletic trainer?**

Certification by the National Athletic Trainer's Association, American Red Cross, Advanced First Aid and Basic Cardiopulmonary Life Support.

❏❏ **What type of physician specialty is best suited to the care of athletes?**

A primary care physician (family physician, internist, pediatrician and emergency medicine physician) is appropriate for elementary and high school sports. At the amateur, Olympic and professional level, a specialist (orthopedist) may serve the elite athlete alone or in conjunction with a generalist/ primary care physician.

❏❏ **What are the responsibilities of the coaching staff?**

1. Coordination of the athletic program.
2. Assure that all players are cleared for participation.
3. Ensure proper followup on deficiencies before playability is established.
4. Participate in the organization of the preparticipation evaluation.
5. Assumption of athletic trainer duties (prevention and first aid) if there is no trainer available.
6. Maintenance of an optimal sports and playing environment, including nutrition, safety, officiating, conditioning, weight and body composition, athletic facilities and equipment.

❏❏ **Identify the requirements for the team physician.**

1. Medical degree (MD or DO).
2. Unrestricted license to practice medicine and surgery in the state of record.
3. BLS certification.
4. Working knowledge of sports emergency and trauma care including management of musculoskeletal injuries and general medical conditions.

5. Strong motivation.
6. Excellent communication skills.
7. Availability.

❑❑ What other credentials are desirable for a team physician?

1. Regular CME in sports medicine.
2. ACLS/ PALS.
3. ATLS.
4. Membership and participation in a sports medicine society.
5. Involvement in academic sports medicine.
6. Knowledge base in compensation, disability and medicolegal issues.
7. Board certification in specialty.
8. Fellowship training and certification in sports medicine.
9. Involvement in a sporting activity of choice.

❑❑ What are the administrative responsibilities of the team physician?

1. Definition of the roles of the members of the sports medicine team.
2. Establishment of a chain of command.
3. Emergency drill planning and training.
4. Event coverage protocols.
5. Assessment of the adequacy of environmental / playing conditions.
6. Equipment/supply assessments.
7. Regular education of and communication with athletes, staff, families, colleagues and community (press).
8. Malpractice and medicolegal policies and protocols.

❑❑ What are the clinical responsibilities of the position?

1. Confidential preparticipation screening and clearance
2. Event coverage including on and off field management of injuries, rehabilitation and return to play
3. Assurance of proper medical record documentation and security
4. Provision of appropriate preventive counseling and education
5. Coordination of all aspects of the sports medicine team

❑❑ Who is responsible for the first aid knowledge of the coaching staff?

The team physician.

❑❑ Identify the important equipment and supplies for the sports medicine team.

The training room (Athletic Medical Unit) must have a separate area with controlled access in which is kept a crash kit for CPR and a sports medicine bag which is maintained by the athletic trainer.

❑❑ What is the most important criteria for success as a team physician?

Professional autonomy with respect to all clinical decisions.

❏❏ **Does a physician's malpractice policy cover him at " away " games?**

The answer depends on the medical malpractice insurance carrier and the location of the game (in state vs out of state).

❏❏ **Is the team physician an employee of the school where he is a team doctor?**

Usually not, since the position of the team physician is typically non salaried or *pro bono*. However, a signed contract or agreement is a good idea since it defines the respective roles of the physician, trainer, coach and school officials.

❏❏ **Who normally supervises the sports related health care needs of the athletes?**

The trainer.

❏❏ **When is the team physician in charge?**

Whenever he / she is present.

❏❏ **When an athlete is injured on the playing field, who goes out to make the initial assessment?**

In most states the trainer operates under physician directed protocols only. Thus, the injured athlete on the field is the patient of the supervising physician, regardless of whether or not the physician is on the playing field. In practice, the trainer goes out first since most injuries are minor and parental apprehension is minimized. If the physician is needed, a prepared signal is used. Once on the playing field, the physician assumes direct care.

❏❏ **Review the on field evaluation steps.**

ABC's and assessment of the extent of the injury, followed by removal from the field if the injury is determined not to be life threatening in order for further evaluation to occur. It is unwise to determine the disposition of an athlete when the area of injury is incompletely exposed. Life threatening injuries should be expeditiously stabilized and rapidly transported to the nearest emergency facility.

❏❏ **Who should accompany the athlete with a life threatening injury?**

The team physician. The team physician for the opposing team should be called upon to serve both teams during the remainder of the game.

❏❏ **Who has final authority on injuries and playability of an athlete?**

The team physician.

❏❏ **Who is responsible for followup?**

The team physician.

MEDICAL SCIENCE

ANATOMY AND BIOMECHANICS

GENERAL ANATOMY

☐☐ Name the three cardinal planes of the body.

Transverse, frontal (coronal) and sagittal.

ARM, ELBOW AND SHOULDER

☐☐ What is the normal resting position of the scapula on the rib cage?

The spine of the scapula usually is located at T-4 and the inferior pole is located at T-7.

☐☐ What muscle in the shoulder girdle is most active (fires continuously at the highest level of intensity) throughout the throwing process?

Serratus Anterior.

☐☐ Why does the serratus anterior muscle fire continuously during throwing?

The serratus anterior is needed to move the scapula to the appropriate location and then to fix the scapula to the back of the chest wall so that the lever arm of the glenohumeral joint can perform its function without wobbling.

☐☐ What two muscles or muscle groups are responsible for keeping the humerus in the glenoid socket after release of a ball with throwing?

Biceps (long head) and the Rotator Cuff (supraspinatus, infraspinatus, teres minor, and subscapularis).

☐☐ Which of these two muscle groups has the final responsibility for ensuring that the humerus maintains its integrity with the glenoid socket?

Long head of the biceps.

☐☐ What is the main muscle involved in the final acceleration of the arm during throwing?

Triceps (extension of the elbow).

❏❏ **How does the body prevent the elbow from going into forceful hyperextension after release of the ball?**

By engaging the biceps in an eccentric fashion.

❏❏ **During the musculoskeletal screening of the preparticipation physical examination, what three signs of serratus anterior weakness may be apparent to the examiner when viewing the athlete's back?**

Winging of the scapula off the back of chest wall; inferior pole of the scapula depressed below other scapula (usually sits at T7); scapula is protracted (further away from vertebral spines than unaffected side - because an injured muscle shortens in length).

❏❏ **Which head of the biceps is responsible for the forceful concentric contractions associated with strength training when the elbow is flexed toward the shoulder?**

Short head which attaches at the coracoid process.

❏❏ **From the point in the overhand throwing motion when the arm is fully cocked (momentarily stationary), how much speed or force (angular momentum) is generated during the ensuing milliseconds as the arm explodes forward to release the ball? You may answer in degrees per second or revolutions of the arm per second.**

7200 degrees per second (20 revolutions per second).

❏❏ **Which two specific muscles are responsible for abducting your arm to 90 degrees?**

Deltoid and supraspinatus. The deltoid has main responsibility for motion during the first 60 degrees, and the supraspinatus for next 30 degrees.

❏❏ **Which muscle is supposed to fire first in initiating pure abduction of the shoulder?**

Supraspinatus. Although the deltoid is the primary mover of the arm in abduction for the first 60 degrees, the supraspinatus (and the infraspinatus and the subscapularis) must contract first or simultaneously to ensure that the direction of motion of the humerus is in a rotational fashion and not linear (translational).

❏❏ **What pathological condition(s) arise(s) when the deltoid fires before the supraspinatus during shoulder abduction and why?**

Impingement and bursitis. Unopposed deltoid firing results in the translational movement of the humerus upward in the glenoid socket. Raising of the humeral head thus reduces the already limited available space for the supraspinatus tendon under the acromial arch of the scapula. As the supraspinatus belatedly contracts, the tendon may face compressive forces between the under surface of the acromion process and the humeral head. This friction force may affect the bursa or tendon.

❑❑ **What does the body "automatically" do to minimize or prevent the deltoid muscle from overwhelming the supraspinatus muscle during the initial phases of shoulder abduction (as described in the question above)?**

Simultaneous and equal co-contractions of the subscapularis and infraspinatus/teres minor muscles whenever the deltoid contracts. This action of the force couple stabilizes the humerus in the glenoid socket, specifically resisting the upward translational action of unopposed deltoid contraction. With the humeral head firmly in the glenoid socket, contraction of the supraspinatus will produce a pure rotational movement in initiating abduction, reducing the likelihood of creating shoulder impingement or bursitis.

❑❑ **Name the extrinsic muscles of the shoulder girdle that insert on the scapula.**

Latissimus dorsi, serratus anterior, pectoralis minor, trapezius, rhomboids, levator scapulae.

❑❑ **Name the intrinsic muscles of the shoulder girdle.**

Rotator cuff muscles (supraspinatus, infraspinatus, teres minor, and subscapularis), Deltoid muscle (three leaves - anterior, middle and posterior).

❑❑ **Name the six pure movements of the glenohumeral joint.**

Abduction, horizontal adduction, forward flexion, backward extension, internal rotation, external rotation.

❑❑ **What three movement patterns can be used to quickly measure the range of motion of the six pure movements of the glenohumeral joint?**

1. Touch the opposite shoulder in front (forward flexion and horizontal adduction);
2. Touch the opposite shoulder in back [crossing behind your head]; external rotation and abduction; 3. Place your thumb as far up your back as you can (extension and internal rotation).

❑❑ **In a very large portion of the population, there will be asymmetry in the level of placing the thumb up the back (highest spine reached). Is the lesser range of motion commonly in the dominant arm or the non-dominant arm?**

The dominant arm is the arm that usually demonstrates this decreased range of motion in extension and internal rotation. While the athlete will consider their dominant arm as the superior extremity, this lack of motion is not an asset. Full range of motion is required for optimal performance, especially in throwing activities.

❑❑ **Does the presence of decreased extension and internal rotation in the glenohumeral joint of the shoulder in the *asymptomatic* athlete carry any clinical significance?**

Yes it does. In a large study of tennis athletes, those asymptomatic athletes with decreased range of motion were at higher risk for shoulder injury than those with equal range of both glenohumeral joints when followed prospectively over a season. If coupled with evidence of problems with scapula stabilization (weak serratus anterior muscle), the chances of injury were even higher.

❏❏ **Which muscle is responsible for scapular retraction (making the shoulder blades meet in the midline)?**

Rhomboids.

❏❏ **Which muscle is mainly responsible for scapular protraction (wrapping your arms around yourself, giving yourself a hug)?**

Serratus anterior primarily with a little help from the pectorals.

❏❏ **During full abduction of the shoulder (bringing your hands from your sides to meet directly overhead), at what point in the arc does clavicular elevation play a role?**

Above the horizontal - after 90 degrees of abduction.

❏❏ **During full abduction of the shoulder (the arm part of the "jumping jack"), in which the hand has moved through an arc of 180 degrees, what percentage of this movement is attributable to scapula upward rotation and what percent to glenohumeral rotational movement?**

Glenohumeral 67% (120 degrees) and Scapular rotation 33% (60 degrees).

❏❏ **Where is the single point attachment of the shoulder girdle to the axial skeleton?**

The sternoclavicular joint (SC) at the sternum.

❏❏ **The strongest anatomic structure in the entire shoulder girdle (from the fingertips to the sternoclavicular joint) is what? In other words, if one fell on an outstretched hand and arm, which anatomic structure is least likely to be injured?**

The sternoclavicular (SC) joint. Therefore, one is more likely to fracture, dislocate or sprain the many bones and ligaments in the hand, wrist, forearm, elbow, upper arm, shoulder and clavicle than to sprain the joint that holds the shoulder girdle to the axial skeleton.

❏❏ **What important anatomic structures are at high risk for damage with a posterior sprain/dislocation of the sternoclavicular (SC) joint?**

The subclavian artery - as well as the subclavian vein, trachea and esophagus.

❏❏ **Hypertrophy of which neck muscle is associated with one type of thoracic outlet syndrome?**

Scalene hypertrophy causes compression of the nerve roots as they traverse to form the brachial plexus.

❏❏ **Name the two types of cartilage found in joints such as the shoulder or knee.**

Articular cartilage and fibrocartilage.

❏❏ **In the elbow, which forearm bone articulates with the capitellum of the humerus?**

The head of the radius.

❏❏ **In the elbow, describe the location of the wrist flexors and extensors.**

The wrist flexors originate on the medial side of the elbow, at the medial epicondyle of the humerus and near the ulna; these muscles insert on the palmar side of the wrist, hand and fingers. The wrist extensors originate on the lateral side of the elbow, at the lateral epicondyle of the humerus and near the radius; these muscles insert on the dorsal side of the wrist, hand and fingers.

❏❏ **Name the five nerves that are derived from the brachial plexus.**

Musculocutaneous, radial, ulnar, median and axillary nerves.

❏❏ **What is the shape of the proximal end of the radius bone?**

Circular, with a "fan-belt" like ligamentous attachment to the underlying structures. This shape and ligamentous restraint permits smooth pronation and supination of the wrist from the elbow region. In young children, when pulled by the arm, it is possible to sublux the radial head from its surrounding ligament. A simple rotational maneuver restores the proper anatomy.

WRIST AND HAND

❏❏ **Which wrist bone serve as the "keystone" of the two rows of bones?**

The lunate.

❏❏ **Which wrist bone is most commonly injured during a fall on an outstretched hand?**

The navicular (or scaphoid) bone. This bone is vulnerable to injury since it bears direct force of impact. . It receives limited blood supply with the flow coming from the distal end toward the proximal end. Thus fractures through the middle of the bone can cut-off blood supply. Immediate radiological diagnosis is difficult. Although fractured, the navicular bone may not show plain x-ray changes for several weeks. A complication of this injury is a non-union, with the fracture failing to heal itself because of its unusual and limited blood supply.

❑❑ **How is the navicular bone readily located on physical examination?**

The navicular sits just below the base of the thumb (abutting the radial head). As one extends the thumb, the two extensor tendons of the thumb become visible. The space between the wrist joint line and these two tendons forms the "anatomic snuff box". The navicular bone is palpated by pressing between the two tendons just distal to the radial head.

❑❑ **Name the carpal bones of the wrist.**

Navicular (scaphoid), lunate, triquetrum, pisiform - first proximal row [radius to ulna]
Trapezium, trapezoid, capitellum, hamate - second distal row [radius to ulna].

❑❑ **Name the three main nerves that innervate the hand and fingers.**

The ulnar, median and radial nerves.

❑❑ **Describe the spinal segment origins for the radial, median and ulnar nerves.**

These nerves arise from the terminal branches of the brachial plexus and have motor and sensory components. Ulnar C8, T1; Median C6,C7,C8,T1, Radial C5,C6,C7, C8, T1.

❑❑ **Describe the cutaneous sensory innervation of the palmar surface of the wrist and hand.**

Ulnar nerve - 5th finger and palm and medial half of 4th (ring) finger.
Median nerve -   entire palm from lateral half of ring finger to thumb and wrist except for lateral area by thumb.
Radial nerve -   lateral portion of thumb only.

❑❑ **Describe the cutaneous sensory innervation of the dorsal surface on the wrist and hand.**

Ulnar nerve - 5th finger and half of 4th finger plus outer half of dorsum of hand and wrist.
Median nerve - 2nd, 3rd fingers from middle of proximal phalanx distally; 4th finger side and thumb medial (inner) side.
Radial nerve -   inner half of dorsum, 2nd, 3rd fingers to middle of proximal phalanx, and thumb lateral (outer) side.

HIP AND KNEE

❑❑ **What is "natural" location for the patella?**

The patella rests in the intracondylar groove of the distal femur. This location is above the joint line between the tibia and fibula. The patella is encased by the quadriceps tendon.

❏❏ **What are the three common injuries ("the unhappy triad") which occur when an athlete is hit from the lateral side of his knee and driven inwardly?**

Anterior cruciate ligament sprain, medial collateral ligament sprain; and meniscal tear. With meniscal tears, the lateral side affected more often than the medial side.

❏❏ **As the knee flexes, in which direction does the meniscal cartilage move?**

The cartilage moves posteriorly (backward).

❏❏ **Which muscle of the quadriceps group is the first muscle to atrophy following injury and the last to recover during a rehabilitation program?**

The vastus medialis obliquus (VMO). It is the smallest of the visible quadriceps muscles with its muscle belly located most distally. It appears to be large and near the patella, but it is the weakest and most vulnerable muscle of the quad group.

❏❏ **When the quadriceps muscles contract, which muscle applies medial forces and which muscles lateral vector forces?**

The vastus medialis (VMO) pulls medially, the rectus femoris and vastus lateralis pull laterally. The lateral force vectors are much stronger than the medial force vector, tending to draw the patella laterally.

❏❏ **What are the three anatomic landmarks that determine the "Q" or quadriceps angle?**

The anterior iliac crest, the center of the patella and the tibial tubercle on the proximal tibia (where the patellar tendon inserts). Since two points determine a line, the angle of intersection of the two lines created by the joining the center of the patella to the two other points is the Q angle. There continues to be debate about the range of normal and abnormal for males and females. Q angles greater than 20 degrees for males are definitely outside of 2 S.D.

❏❏ **What muscles are located directly behind the knee, occupying the popliteal fossa?**

The head of the gastrocnemius muscle, as well as the plantaris and popliteus.

❏❏ **Name five functions of the knee meniscal cartilage.**

Increases joint congruity, nourishes the articular cartilage of the tibia and femur, provides shock absorption, distributes the pressure from the femur from two points to the entire joint surface, increases the stability of the knee joint.

❏❏ **Name the three muscles that comprise the pes anserinus group which attaches on the medial proximal aspect of the tibia.**

Hamstring (semitendinosus), gracilis and sartorius.

❏❏ **As the sciatic nerve passes through the gluteal region, which muscle has this nerve pass directly through its fibers in a significant percentage of the population? In that situation, "sciatic pain" arises but does not have its origin in the spinal column, vertebral discs, neural foramina or nerve roots. Contraction and spasm of this muscle can cause sciatic symptoms.**

The piriformis muscle.

❏❏ **Describe the origin, pathway and insertion of the iliotibial band (ITB).**

The iliotibial band has its origins in the hip as the tensor fascia lata muscle which courses over the greater trochanter and down the lateral aspect of the femur. This thick band of connective tissue crosses the distal femur by the lateral epicondyle and inserts on the anterior lateral proximal tibia at "Gerdy's tubercle".

❏❏ **What is the test for evaluating the tightness of the iliotibial band?**

The Ober test. The patient lies on his side with his back facing the examiner. The patient brings his back right to the near edge of the examining table. The examiner uses his body to stabilize the patient at the pelvis and grasps the upper leg at the ankle. The hip is extended, and then the knee is lowered toward the examination table. In the normal situation, the knee can easily reach the table or below the table. When the ITB is tight, it cannot reach the level of the table.

❏❏ **What is the anatomic cause for iliotibial band (ITB) friction syndrome?**

When the knee is extended, the ITB sits anterior to the lateral epicondyle; when the knee is flexed, the band becomes located posterior to the epicondyle. [Since two points determine a line, moving of the tibia in relation to the hip during knee flexion mandates migration of the ITB.] The repeated crossing over the lateral epicondyle with repetitive activities such as running can cause irritation to the ITB, unless increases are done gradually, allowing the body to toughen up rather than become irritated and injured.

❏❏ **What is the most common mechanism for injuring the ACL?**

The leg hyperextends, through contact, through landing stiff-legged, through failing to engage the posterior musculature to decelerate the body's movement of the thigh and torso on the tibia.

❏❏ **What are considered to be a pathognomonic signs and symptoms for an ACL injury?**

Immediate pain, hearing or sensing a "pop" sound ("like popping the cork of a champagne bottle"), rapid onset of central knee swelling (even when vigorously applying ice and compression), instability with ambulation.

❏❏ **What is the most common mechanism for injuring the MCL of the knee?**

A blow from the outside driving the tibia and femur medially.

❏❏ **What structures comprise the posterior lateral corner of the knee?**

The lateral collateral ligament (LCL), the posterior cruciate ligament (PCL), the arcuate complex and the popliteus muscle tendon.

❏❏ **Name the six pure planes of movement of the hip joint.**

Forward flexion, abduction, extension, internal rotation, external rotation, horizontal adduction.

❏❏ **During what portion of the range of motion of the knee during extension does the VMO have its maximal effect?**

The last 15 to 20 degrees of forceful extension at the knee, especially when the hip is flexed.

❏❏ **In the knee, which collateral ligament is stronger, the lateral collateral ligament (LCL) or medial collateral ligament (MCL)?**

The MCL is much stronger. The MCL is thick with many fibers. The MCL attaches over a large portion of the distal femur and the proximal tibia, firmly anchored to the bones, enabling itself to resist significant energy generated during a blow to the outside of the knee. This force drives the knee inward and causes the MCL to develop tension. The LCL attaches from the lateral epicondyle to the proximal fibula head; it is strong but relatively thin (like a guitar or violin string).

UPPER AND LOWER BACK

❏❏ **What are the four principal functions of the vertebrae?**

Support (vertebral body), protection of the spinal cord (vertebral arch), limitation of excessive movement to prevent dislocation (articular processes) and body movement (from muscle attachments to the transverse processes and spinous process).

❏❏ **What are the three points of contact between two lumbar vertebrae?**

The vertebral body anteriorly and the two posterior facet joints create a "tripod" formation. The inferior articular processes (pedicles) articulate with the adjacent superior articular processes to form the facet joints. The intervertebral disc rests between the vertebral bodies (which are stacked up like a series of spools of thread).

❏❏ **What is the difference in the shape of the vertebral bodies between the thoracic vertebrae and the lumbar and cervical vertebrae?**

The lumbar and cervical vertebral bodies have transverse diameters greater than anterior-posterior (AP) diameters, while the opposite is found in the thoracic vertebrae.

❏❏ **What is the shape of the vertebral foramina in the cervical region, the thoracic region and the lumbar region?**

The lumbar and cervical regions have triangular foramina and the thoracic region has circular foramina.

❏❏ **What is weakest anatomic location in each lumbar vertebra?**

The pars intra-articularis.

❏❏ **What are the two main anatomic features of the intervertebral discs?**

The liquid center and the rings of the annulus fibrosis.

❏❏ **How many points of contact exist between two cervical vertebrae, and does this differ from the arrangement seen in the thoracic and lumbar regions?**

In addition to the common tripod formations consisting of the posterior elements (paired facet joints) and the vertebral body, there are two uncovertebral joints, also known as the joints of Luschka. These joints arise along the superior lateral margins of the vertebral bodies as lip-like projections on C3 through C7.

❏❏ **How do the first two cervical vertebrae differ from the others?**

The first vertebra is known as the atlas for its ring shape and absence of transverse processes or spines. The shape of the vertebral foramina of the atlas is pear-like, with the anterior opening permitting the odontoid process of the second vertebra ("axis") to occupy that space. This allows for head rotation and nodding movements. Further, both the atlas and axis do not have a true vertebral body.

❏❏ **In which direction does the liquid center of the intervertebral disc generally move when one sits for a long time and loses the natural lordotic curve in the lumbar spine?**

The liquid center is directed posteriorly, increasing the chances for low back pain. As the liquid center is forced in a single direction for excessive periods of time, the integrity of the annulus fibrosis is compromised, progressively leading to the pathological stages of prolapse, then herniation and then frank rupture of the liquid center.

❏❏ **Name the six pure planes of movement of the cervical and lumbar spines.**

Flexion, extension, rotation left and right, side-bend left and side-bend right.

❏❏ **What are the names for the connective tissue that cover the anterior and posterior surface of the vertebral bodies?**

The anterior longitudinal ligament and the posterior longitudinal ligament. The anterior longitudinal ligament is comprised of broad, strong, fibrous bands. The posterior longitudinal ligament is a taut but somewhat flimsy band passing from disc to disc. Behind the vertebral body, the ligament is narrow and serves to smoothen the anterior wall of the vertebral canal. Behind each disc, however, the ligament fans out and takes on a diamond shape, where it sends off fibers and receives fibers.

❏❏ **What is the name of the connective tissue that covers the anterior portion of the facet joints (the vertebral arches)?**

The ligamentum flavum.

❏❏ **What two purposes do the transverse processes and vertebral spines serve?**

They serve as sites of origins (and insertions) for spinal muscles and ligaments. They also provide physical protection for the spinal cord that traverses through the vertebral foramina.

❏❏ **In the low back, starting from the spinous process and moving laterally, name the six deep major muscles of the back.**

The *interspinalis* muscle attaches to the lateral margin of the spinous process; the *multifidus* muscle attaches more laterally, arising from the spinous process and vertebral arch. Even more laterally lies the *longissimus* muscle and then the *iliocostalis* muscle, both arising from the posterior border of the transverse processes. The most lateral muscle is the *quadratus lumborum muscle*, which attaches near the tip (posterior inferior lateral margin) of the transverse process. The *psoas* muscle lies anterior medial to the quadratus lumborum and its medial margin attaches to the vertebral body.

Sandwiched between these major muscles, the *intertransversarius* muscles run from transverse process to transverse process, along with a ligamentous covering.

❏❏ **In the lower extremity, which spinal segments are responsible for the knee jerk reflex and the Achilles/ankle reflex.**

Knee jerk - L4-L5; Ankle/knee jerk - L5-S1.

LEG, ANKLE AND FOOT

❏❏ **Name the four pure planes of movement of the ankle.**

Plantarflexion, dorsiflexion. Inversion and eversion.

❏❏ **Name the two muscles that support the medial transverse arch in the foot.**

Anterior tibialis and posterior tibialis.

❏❏ **Where does the peroneus brevis muscle insert in the foot and what is its function?**

At the base of the fifth metatarsal; it is the principal everter of the foot.

❑❑ **Where does the peroneus longus muscle insert? By which bones in the foot does it change course?**

On the first metatarsal bone. It changes course twice, first by the distal fibula and again as it traverses the cuboid bone on its way to its attachment on the first ray.

❑❑ **Name the structure in the foot that supports the longitudinal arch.**

The plantar fascia, which originates on the calcaneus and inserts are the distal ends of the five rays.

❑❑ **Name the term commonly used to describe the ligamentous attachment of the anterior distal tibia and fibula at the ankle mortise. What is the term used when this ligament is injured enough to partially separate the bones.**

Syndesmosis; the injury is a diastasis of the syndesmosis.

❑❑ **In assessing ankle function following an ankle injury, what function of the ankle is often weeks and months behind the others in recovery?**

Proprioception (position sense or balance). The inversion mechanism of injury can also damage nerves, decreasing proprioception. Full resolution may not occur for several months. Exercises to promote proprioception are an important component of an ankle rehab program.

❑❑ **What anatomic position is the ankle in during most inversion injuries?**

Plantarflexion and inversion.

❑❑ **What is the anatomic position of the ankle during most eversion injuries? How does the injury typically occur?**

The foot is usually planted on the ground. A force is applied laterally on the distal fibula, driving the medial portion of the ankle (deltoid ligament) inwardly. One example of this mechanism occurs when one basketball player is waiting for a rebound and another player lands on their planted leg.

❑❑ **What three significant injuries can occur from this eversion mechanism injury to the ankle?**

Sprain of the medial deltoid ligament, widening on diastasis of the syndesmosis (anterior tibiofibular ligament), and fracture of the distal fibula. It is of interest to note that the most painful of the three injuries is the medial ligament sprain, the only one of the three for which surgery is NOT needed! Accordingly, always palpate the distal fibula and anterior tibiofibular ligament whenever the eversion mechanism occurs.

❑❑ **Which compartment of the lower leg, containing which muscles, is most susceptible to compartment syndrome and why?**

The anterior compartment, located just lateral to the tibia is most vulnerable because it is contained in a fibrous sheath with limited capacity for expansion for increased blood flow associated with intense athletic activity. The anterior tibialis muscle and the dorsiflexors of the foot and ankle are part of this muscle group.

❏❏ **Which lower leg bone, the tibia or fibula, extends more distally?**

The fibula, making the lateral malleolus relatively longer and providing bony stability to the lateral portion of the ankle mortise joint.

❏❏ **In the normal calcaneus, how many degrees of inversion and eversion motion is there in the range of motion?**

The heel inverts 30 degrees and everts 15 degrees.

❏❏ **Which lower leg muscle engages when running downhill but not when running on level ground?**

Popliteus.

❏❏ **In the ankle, which ligament complex is stronger, the medial deltoid ligament or the lateral ligaments (anterior talofibular, calcaneofibular, posterior talofibular, and anterior tibiofibular ligament)? Give several reasons for your selection.**

The medial deltoid ligament complex. In part because the tibia does not extend as far distally as the fibula and in part because the body generally must protect from external forces from the outside driving the body inwardly (valgus stress), the ligaments on the medial side of a joint tend to be stronger. The deltoid ligament is comprised of multiple strips of connective tissue forming a dense triangle (hence the name deltoid); the lateral ligaments by comparison are thin and flimsy strips of tissue.

❏❏ **Name the two large tarsal bones and the five small tarsal bones, from medial to lateral. Describe how these bones articulate with each other.**

The two large bones form the rearfoot and the five small bones comprise the midfoot. The calcaneus and talus compose the large bones, with the talus resting atop the calcaneus. The tarsal navicular (medially) and the cuboid (laterally) articulate in the talonavicular and calcaneocuboid joints. Distal to the navicular bone, the medial (1st) cuneiform, middle (2nd) cuneiform and lateral (3rd) cuneiform articulate with the navicular. The lateral cuneiform articulates laterally with the cuboid.

❏❏ **How does the body accomplish the task of altering the line of force for the peroneus brevis muscle? This muscle originates at the proximal fibula and runs vertically down the leg. Its tendon inserts at the base of the fifth metatarsal. When the muscle contracts, it everts the foot.**

Various connective tissue formations (called retinacula) create "staple-like" arches over the tendon to keep it within its anatomic track when the peroneus brevis muscle contracts. Through this series of arches, the direction of force of the tendon is altered from the vertical plane to the horizontal plane.

BIOMECHANICS

❏❏ **Which factor is of greater significance in creating energy during a collision between two athletes, mass or speed?**

Speed. The kinetic energy equals 1/2 the mass times velocity squared. (KE= $1/2mv^2$).

❏❏ **Name the two phases of the walking gait cycle.**

In walking, one foot is always on the ground; about 20% of the time, both feet are on the ground. The foot touching the ground is in the *stance phase*; the other leg is in the *swing phase*. The gait cycle is measured from heel strike on one foot until the next heel strike of the same foot.

❏❏ **Name the elements of the stance phase of the walking gait cycle.**

The stance phase begins with *contact* at heel strike (just as the other leg is lifting off from toe-off into swing phase); in heel strike, the foot is ahead of the body. The foot moves from a supinated position at heel strike through pronation to achieve foot flat at *mid-stance* (as the body moves directly over the foot). After the body passes over the planted foot, heel rise occurs beginning *propulsion*, which culminates in toe-off.

❏❏ **Name the elements of the swing phase of the gait cycle.**

The swing phase leg moves backward just after toe-off, then swings forward, and finally descends toward the ground for the next heel strike. These are termed acceleration, midswing and deceleration, respectively. The swing phase takes place entirely during mid-stance (foot flat).

❏❏ **Describe the phases of the walking gait cycle when both feet are in contact with the ground.**

During contact and propulsion. Heel strike begins on one leg just after heel rise begins on the other. Foot flat (the start of mid-stance) is achieved just after toe-off is completed.

❏❏ **What proportion of the time is the leg in each portion of the stance phase during the gait cycle?**

Contact 25%, mid-stance 40% and propulsion 35%.

❏❏ **Describe the normal pathway of the weight-bearing ground reactive force during the stance phase.**

Heel contact occurs over the lateral heel at heel strike and moves toward the arch and toes; during mid-stance, the force vector angles across the arch toward the head of the first metatarsal. At heel rise, the beginning of propulsion, the weight is under the first MP joint. The vector proceeds through the great toe at toe-off.

❑❑ For muscles such as the biceps and quadriceps, where in the range of motion is the greatest torque forces generated and why? Choices include at the ends of the range of motion (near full flexion or full extension) or in the middle of the range of motion.

The greatest torque forces are commonly generated in the middle of the range of motion. In part, this is related to the geometry of the joints, whereby the force generated is related to the sine function of the angle. Since the sine of 0° and 180° are zero and the sine of 90° is 1, contractions near the midrange of joints will generate the highest forces.

❑❑ In neck motion as well as shoulder girdle motion, for example, what is a key principle of movement the body employs?

Use of force couples, the synchronized and coordinated contraction of several muscles to achieve motion. In some cases, some muscles act as stabilizers while others provide dynamic forces to cause bones to move smoothly toward or away from each other (co-contraction). In other situations, agonists contract concentrically to cause parts to move toward each other while antagonists contract eccentrically to subtly resist unopposed agonist action.

❑❑ During fine motor activities involving little motion but delicate action, how does the body achieve such control?

Through co-contractions, whereby agonist and antagonist muscles contract together in almost equal amounts to produce a stabilizing effect with only a slight differential, resulting in delicate fine motor "motionless" activities.

❑❑ When a figure skater does a spin initially with arms extended, how much more rapidly does she spin when she brings her arms down to her side?

A three-fold increase in her angular momentum.

❑❑ The biceps and sartorius muscles are examples of what mechanical type of muscle?

A two joint muscle, crossing joints proximally and distally. The biceps crosses the shoulder and elbow joints; the sartorius crosses the hip and knee joint.

❑❑ Describe the three types of levers noted in physics. Which is the most commonly used in the body for movement?

In the first class of lever, force is applied at one end and the resistance to be overcome is at the other end; the fulcrum or pivot point is in the middle (such as a seesaw). In the second class of lever, force is applied at one end, but the resistance is located above the fulcrum or pivot (such as a crowbar under a tree stump). In the third class of lever, force is exerted between the pivot point and the resistance. This is the most common lever system used in the body. For example, if we hold an object in our hand and wish to bring it toward our shoulder, through contraction of the biceps muscle, whose attachment is on the forearm proximal to the hand, this task is accomplished.

❏❏ **In regard to mechanical stress placed on the spinal column while holding objects, what is difference in load factor when an object is hugged closely to the body versus held out at arms length?**

Approximately a two-fold difference in load factor.

HEAD AND NECK

❏❏ **When examining the cervical vertebrae, which spinous prominence is most visible?**

C-7, also referred to as vertebra prominens.

❏❏ **Describe the curves of the spinal column as seen from a sagittal section.**

In the cervical and lumbar regions, a lordotic curve is present; in the thoracic region, a kyphotic curve exists.

❏❏ **In assessing head, neck and shoulder posture, what landmarks are used?**

Examining from the side of the patient (in a sagittal view), the neck should maintain its lordotic curve and the shoulders should be held upright and the scapulae somewhat retracted. In poor posture, the neck loses its lordotic curve and protrudes forward, while the shoulder are rounded and stooped forward (with scapulae protraction). In proper erect posture, if a plumb line is dropped from the earlobe, it should bisect the acromium process and pass over the greater trochanter.

❏❏ **From which cervical nerve roots does the long thoracic nerve originate and what key muscle does it innervate?**

The long thoracic nerve arises from the plexus roots of C5-C6-C7 and it innervates the serratus anterior muscle.

❏❏ **Describe the origin and insertion of the pectoralis major muscle and its primary action.**

The pectoralis major has a crescent shaped origin, arising along the sternum, proximal clavicle and the 5th and/or 6th costal cartilages; it inserts on the anterior/lateral aspect of the proximal humerus (lateral to the insertions of the teres major and latissimus dorsi muscles). Its action is to adduct the humerus toward the midline.

❏❏ **Describe the origin and insertion of the pectoralis minor muscle.**

The pectoralis minor muscle arises from the 3rd, 4th and 5th ribs (may also have an origin on the 2nd and 6th ribs). The pectoralis minor muscle inserts on the coracoid process, just medial to the origin of the short head of the biceps and coraco-brachialis muscles.

❏❏ **Name the two ligaments which secure the distal end of the clavicle to the scapula.**

The acromioclavicular ligament (AC) and the coracoclavicular ligament (CC).

❏❏ **Name the three columns of the deep muscles of the back that comprise the erector spinae (sacrospinalis).**

The spinalis, longissimus and iliocostalis.

❏❏ **Which of the three muscles of the deep muscles of the back extends all the way to the skull to insert into the mastoid process?**

The longissimus.

❏❏ **Name the muscles in the five layers of the upper back, starting from the superficial and working deeper.**

Layer 1: Trapezius and latissimus dorsi.
Layer 2: Levator scapulae and rhomboids.
Layer 3: Serratus posterior superior.
Layer 4: Splenius capitis and cervicis.
Layer 5: Erector spinae - spinalis, longissimus and iliocostalis.

❏❏ **As the subclavian artery emerges from between the clavicle and the first rib, behind which muscle does it pass?**

The scalenus anterior muscle. The subclavian artery courses between the scalenus anterior and scalenus medius muscle as it crosses anterior to the first rib.

❏❏ **Which spinal segments innervate the anterior scalene muscle?**

C3, C4, C5, with C4 being the primary segment.

❏❏ **What are the margins of the anterior triangle of the neck?**

The anterior triangle is bounded by the sternocleidomastoid muscle, the median line of the neck and the lower border of the mandible.

❏❏ **What are the margins of the posterior triangle of the neck?**

The posterior triangle is bounded by the trapezius muscle, the sternocleidomastoid muscle and the middle third of the clavicle.

❏❏ **Name the origin and insertion of the scalene anterior?**

The scalene anterior muscle originates at the anterior tubercles of the transverse processes of the 2nd through 6th cervical vertebrae and inserts on the lateral portion of the first rib at the scalene tubercle and cranial crest.

MEDICAL SCIENCE

GROWTH AND DEVELOPMENT

❏❏ **Define growth.**

Growth is an increase in the size of a body as a whole or the size attained by specific parts of the body.

❏❏ **What three cellular processes underlie the changes in size which define growth?**

Growth is the combination of an increase in cell number (hyperplasia), an increase in cell size (hypertrophy) and an increase in intercellular substances (accretion).

❏❏ **Define maturation. How does maturation differ from growth?**

Maturation refers to the tempo and timing of progress toward the mature biological state. Growth focuses on size while maturation focuses on progress in, or rate of, attaining size.

❏❏ **Define development.**

In the biological context, development is the differentiation of cells along specialized lines of function. Most of this biological differentiation of development takes place prenatally. The second context is behavioral and relates to the development of competence in a variety of interrelated domains as the child adjusts to his or her cultural milieu. Examples include development of social competence, intellectual or cognitive competence, and emotional competence ("well-being"). Within the context of physical activity, one of the major developmental tasks of childhood is the development and refinement of skillful performance in a variety of physical activities.

❏❏ **Up through what age is the body developing the basic movement patterns of running, walking and jumping?**

During the first five or six years of life, the development depends largely on the individual's rate of neuromuscular maturation. Only after these basic movement patterns have been established do experience, learning and practice become significant factors in affecting motor competence.

❏❏ **Name the common chronological age periods from childhood through adulthood.**

Infancy comprises the first year of life and is characterized as a period of rapid growth in most bodily systems and dimensions plus rapid development of the neuromuscular system. The average child triples body weight during the first year of life. Childhood spans from the end of infancy to the start of adolescence. Early childhood comprises ages 1 through 5 and middle childhood from age 6 to the onset of adolescence. Adolescence is difficult to define in terms of age, due to the variation of its onset and termination. For girls, the ages range from 8 to 19 and in boys from 10 to 22. During adolescence, most bodily systems become adult structurally and functionally.

❑❑ What structural and functional changes demarcate adolescence?

Structurally, adolescence begins with an acceleration in the rate of growth in stature ("growth spurt"). This rate of structural growth reaches a peak (peak height velocity - PVH), begins a slower or decelerative phase, and finally terminates with the attainment of adult stature. Functionally, adolescence is usually viewed in terms of sexual maturation, which actually begins with changes in the neuroendocrine systems prior to overt physical changes and terminates with the attainment of mature reproductive function.

❑❑ What is the shape of the general growth curve ("Growth Chart") and what are the four phases?

The general growth curve is S-shaped or sigmoid. The four phases are the rapid growth of infancy and early childhood; the steady constant growth of early childhood, the rapid growth during the adolescent growth spurt, and the slow increase and eventual cessation of growth after adolescence.

❑❑ What is the shape of the neural growth curve?

The neural curve characterizes the growth of the brain, nervous system and associated structures, such as the eyes, upper face, and parts of the skull. These tissues experience rapid growth early in postnatal life, so that about 95% of the total increment in size are attained by about 7 years of age. Neural tissues show a steady gain after 7 years of age with a slight growth spurt during adolescence.

❑❑ What is the shape of the genital growth curve?

The genital growth curve characterizes the pattern of primary and secondary sexual characteristics. Genital tissues show slight growth in infancy, followed by a latent period during most of childhood. Genital tissues then experience extremely rapid growth and maturation during their adolescent spurt.

❑❑ What is the shape of the lymphoid curve?

The lymphoid curve describes the growth of the lymph glands, thymus gland, tonsils, appendix and lymphoid patches of tissue in the intestine. These tissues are involved in the child's developing immunological capacities, including resistance to infectious diseases. Lymphoid tissue shows rapid development during infancy and childhood, reaching a maximum at about 11 to 13 years of age. At these ages, children have about twice the lymphoid tissues as they will have as adults. The decline of the lymphoid curve during the second decade of life is related to the involution (shrinking) of the thymus and tonsils at this time.

❏❏ **How does phenotype differ from genotype?**

An individual's genetic makeup, or genotype, can be viewed as his or her potential. The child's physical and physiological characteristics represent his or her observable characteristics, or phenotype. The phenotype is a product of the genotype and environments in which the child is reared.

❏❏ **What are some key factors that determine whether the phenotype approximates genotypic potential?**

The most important factor in the regulation of growth and maturation is probably nutrition. Regular physical exercise plays a role, but so do socioeconomic conditions, hygiene and physical environment.

❏❏ **Body mass index is an important measurement used for determining the relationship between weight and stature. What is the formula used for calculating body mass index?**

Body mass index = weight/stature^2 where weight is expressed in kilograms and stature in meters.

❏❏ **By what age do girls have a faster resting heart rate than boys?**

From 10 years old through adolescence.

❏❏ **The best method for protecting the throwing arm of young baseball pitchers includes what controls on unlimited throwing?**

Counting pitches and establishing a maximum number of pitches per game (based on age and experience); limiting the number of games pitched in (on ALL teams) per week; focusing on fastballs and change-ups exclusively prior to puberty; gradual introduction of curve balls and other breaking pitches after the onset of puberty.

❏❏ **In trying to protect the throwing arms of young baseball pitchers, what are two changes in performance parameters which may indicate impending muscle fatigue?**

Loss of maximal speed and loss of accuracy (control).

❏❏ **During which period of growth and development do girls generally weigh more than boys?**

Generally from ages 9 through 14 years of age.

❏❏ **During which period of growth and development are girls generally taller than boys?**

Generally from ages 9 through 14 years of age.

❑❑ **What are the three basic physique classifications or somatotypes?**

Endomorph, mesomorph and an ectomorph. Endomorphs tend to be "chunky", mesomorphs muscular and "thick" and ectomorphs "thin and reedy". Endomorphy is characterized by predominance of the digestive organs and by softness and roundness of contour throughout the body. Mesomorphy is characterized by predominance of muscle, bone and connective tissue, so that muscles are prominent with sharp definition. Ectomorphy is characterized by linearity and fragility of build, with poor muscle development and a predominance of surface area over body mass.

❑❑ **What is the typical height gain during peak height velocity for boys and girls (cm/yr)?**

Boys 10 cm/yr at age 14 and girls 9 cm/yr at age 12.

❑❑ **What two reasons explain why boys tend to be taller than girls?**

On average, girls begin their pubertal growth spurt two years earlier than boys. During these two years, boys continue to demonstrate the pre-pubertal growth in stature of about 5cm per year. Further, the peak height velocity for boys during their growth spurt is about one cm/yr higher than for girls. On average, girls complete their adult height between ages 15 and 16 and boys between 17 and 18.

❑❑ **To what effect does maternal smoking impact the stature of her offspring?**

Combined effect of smoking during pregnancy and smoking in the home after birth. Stunting of height from smoking: -0.65cm for heavy smokers (>10 cigarettes per day); light smoking (1-9 cigarettes/day) = -.45cm compared to non-smokers. The data was collected on pre-adolescent children, ages 6 to 11 years old.

❑❑ **To what effect, if any, does paternal smoking impact the stature of the offspring?**

Smoking takes places in the home prior to conception and after birth. For heavy smoking father (>10 cigarettes per day) = -0.10cm; for light smoking (1-9 cigarettes per day) = -0.04cm.

❑❑ **What are the six major categories of predisposing medical conditions that contraindicate a player to participate in collision/ contact sports?**

Neurologic, defects in paired systems (i.e. vision, kidneys, testes), organ enlargement, active infections (ie osteomyelitis, pyelonephritis, septic arthritis, boils), vertebropelvic defects, and cardiopulmonary disorders.

❑❑ **What physical findings during the preparticipation physical exam suggest Marfan's syndrome?**

Any male over 6 feet and any female athlete over 5 feet 10 inches in height with two of the following positive findings suggest Marfan's syndrome: cardiac murmur or midsystolic click, kyphoscoliosis, anterior thoracic deformity, arm span greater than height, upper: lower body ratio >1 standard deviation below the mean, myopia, and ectopic lens.

❏❏ **What effect does continued endurance training by the pregnant mother have on the unborn child?**

In a study by Clapp et al, babies born to mothers who continued their exercise regiment throughout their pregnancy consistently had smaller infants, averaging 500 grams lower birth weight.

❏❏ **What effect does continued endurance training by the pregnant mother have on the morbidity of the unborn child?**

A study by Clapp et al showed no increased immediate morbidity of the unborn child.

❏❏ **What is the incidence of fetal alcohol syndrome?**

About 1 in 700 births.

❏❏ **What are the features of an individual born with fetal alcohol syndrome?**

These individuals will present with intrauterine growth retardation (IUGR - "small-for-date"), abnormal facial development, stunted physical growth, microcephaly, and 33% will present with CNS dysfunction.

❏❏ **How are bones formed?**

Intramembranous bone formation develops between embryonic membranes and give rise to bones of the skull. Endochondral bone formation develops from cartilage and gives rise to bones of the postcranial skeleton and even some parts of the cranium.

❏❏ **Name the sections of a growing long bone and describe their activity and function.**

The shaft of the long bone is the diaphysis; it will house the marrow cavity and embryonically generate the growth plate. The cartilaginous growth plate separates the epiphysis and diaphysis. The growth plate itself contains several distinct zones. Nearest the epiphysis (at the distal end of the bone) is the reserve zone; adjacent to that is the zone of cartilage proliferation. Next to that is the zone of cartilage hypertrophy and the elaboration of the intercellular matrix. In this zone of cellular hypertrophy, collagen fibers appear in the intracellular matrix and separate the columns of cartilage cells; the cells hypertrophy and then calcify at the proximal end. The junction of the hypertrophic zone with the diaphysis is called the metaphysis. It is in the metaphysis that actual ossification occurs. Terminal branches of the diaphyseal blood vessels penetrate the cartilage and further erode it. Osteoblasts deposit bone matrix upon the surface remnants of calcified cartilage.

❏❏ **What is the term used to describe the cessation of bony growth?**

Epiphyseal union, when the epiphysis joins the diaphysis directly.

❏❏ **The dry, fat-free skeleton accounts for what percentage of body weight in young infants?**

Three percent of the body weight.

❏❏ **The dry, fat-free skeleton accounts for what percentage of body weight in adults?**

Six to seven percent of the body weight.

❏❏ **Approximately how many muscles are there in the adult body?**

Over 500.

❏❏ **Which muscle type is more prevalent before and shortly after birth in the infant?**

Fast twitch fibers. At birth, about 40% are Type I (slow-twitch fibers), 45% are Type II (fast-twitch fibers) and 15% of fibers are undifferentiated.

❏❏ **As the infant continues to develop, what happens to the motor units of mixed composition?**

By age 1 or 2, muscles containing motor units of mixed composition acquire the properties of slow twitch fibers.

❏❏ **Muscles account for what percentage of the neonate's body weight?**

23%-25%.

❏❏ **Muscles account for what percentage of an adult's body weight?**

40%.

❏❏ **By what age is the male's muscle mass accounting for the greatest percentage of his weight?**

By age 17.7 years, a male's muscle mass accounts for 53.6% of his total weight. By age 20-29 years of age, it accounts for only 51.5% of his weight.

❏❏ **By what age is the female's muscle mass accounting for the greatest percentage of her weight?**

By age 7, a female's muscle mass accounts for 46.6% of her total weight. By age 20-29 years of age, it accounts for only 39.9% of her weight.

❏❏ **What accounts for the brown color in brown fat cells?**

Their distinct color is primarily due to a high concentration of cytochromes and cytochrome enzymes in the mitochondria as well as to a vast vascular supply and hemoglobin content.

❏❏ **What is the function of the foramen ovale during fetal life?**

It served as a temporary one-way valve for blood returning to the right atrium to bypass the right ventricle and flow directly into the left atrium. Thus, much of the fetal blood bypasses the premature lungs. It is estimated only about 10% to 15% of the blood traverses the lungs with each heart contraction.

❏❏ **Name four contributing factors to motor development in the growing child.**

Motor development is a process by which a child acquires movement patterns and skills. The process of neuromuscular maturation, which is probably genetically regulated; the growth and maturity characteristics of the child (size and body composition); the residual effects of prior motor experiences; and new motor experiences per se.

❏❏ **How do the terms motor pattern and motor skill differ?**

A motor pattern is the basic movement involved in the performance of a particular task. Emphasis is on the movements composing the task. Motor skill focuses on the proficiency of completing the task. Motor skill looks at accuracy, precision, and economy of performance.

❏❏ **How do the terms fine motor activity and gross motor activity differ?**

Fine motor refers to movements requiring precision and dexterity, as in manipulative tasks. Gross motor refers to movements of the entire body or major segments of the body, as in locomotor activities. Throwing a ball requires both gross motor and fine motor activity. Speed entails gross motor forces and accuracy and control come from fine motor activity.

❏❏ **What are the three major categories of fundamental movement patterns?**

Locomotor, nonlocomotor, and manipulative. Locomotor refers to patterns in which the body is moving through space (walking, jumping, galloping, hopping, skipping). Nonlocomotor refers to patterns in which specific parts of the body are moved (pushing, pulling, bending, twisting). Manipulative refers to patterns in which objects are moved (throwing, catching, kicking, dribbling, striking, and other activities involving projecting and receiving objects).

❏❏ **Explain how process and product of movement are used to assess fundamental motor patterns and skills.**

When assessing the quality of athletic and physical activity, the process of movement deals with the technique of performing a specific movement in terms of its components (hip rotations, arm action, etc) and specific elements of the activity (angle of takeoff in a jump, length of lever arms, etc). The product of movement concerns the result or outcome of the act (the distance a child jumps, the time elapsed in a dash). In general, but not always, the process and product of a motor performance are related. Good performers in terms of the product usually demonstrate proficiency in the movement process.

☐☐ **In the growing, normally developing infant and young child, what general principles explain attainment of motor abilities?**

Development of motor abilities begins at the head and works down the body to the arms, trunk and legs. With rare exceptions, attainment of skills follows a set sequence and pattern. Although the timing is variable, the order of achievement is predictable. Motor development is viewed as representing the neuromuscular maturation of the child.

☐☐ **By what age should a normally developing child walk independently?**

The child should be able to walk between 11 and 13 months of age. By age 4, the adult walking pattern will be established in most children.

☐☐ **By what age should a normally developing child be able to catch a ball?**

By age 2, the child can catch a ball on an immature level by imitating catching movements. By age 3, the child should be able to catch a ball on an intermediate level.

☐☐ **What are the four developmental categories necessary to catch a ball?**

Initial arm position (preparation); arm movement as the ball approaches; body movement as the ball approaches; and hand positioning and movement in catching the ball. Within each of the four components, there are three to six steps.

☐☐ **What are the four developmental elements necessary to swing a bat?**

(1) Hand grip (the hand nearest the knob of the bat is the same as the foot closest to the pitcher); (2) stance (feet are even and parallel to the side edge of home plate and head turned toward the pitcher); (3) striding forward (lifting the front foot striding toward the pitch resulting in weight transfer from the rear foot to the front foot); and (4) hip rotation (swing begins in the legs, continues through hip rotation and ends with trunk and arm involvement).

☐☐ **What are the biomechanical elements necessary to kick a ball?**

Balancing on the plant leg (forces on the support foot), location of the plant leg immediately adjacent to the ball, angle of approach to the ball, swing limb movement during the backswing and forward swing (flexion at the hip and extension of the knee), ball contact, and follow through.

☐☐ **By what age should a normally developing child be able to skip?**

Girls learn to skip by age 4.5 years of age while boys are able to skip by age 5.

☐☐ **How is an infant's status at birth related to his/her physical development?**

An infant's birth status, particularly birth weight, is an important indicator of his/her physical development. Normal birth weight children tend to physically develop sooner than low birth weigh and premature babies.

How is the development of static strength different in boys and girls?

In girls, static strength improves linearly with age until 16 or 17 years of age with no clear evidence for an adolescent spurt as seen in boys.

How is the development of endurance different in boys and girls?

Similarly, girls do not show an adolescent spurt gain in endurance as seen in boys but sex differences in muscular endurance can actually be noticed by age 8 with boys lasting longer than girls in the flexed horizontal bar test.

What does the shuttle run test measure?

The shuttle run test is used as an indicator of agility, the ability to rapidly change the direction of movement.

How is the development of running speed different in boys and girls?

Boys show a linear improvement in speed from 5 through 17 years of age without clear evidence of an adolescent growth spurt. There is also a linear pattern seen in girls but only from 5 through 12 years of age followed by only a slight increase through age 17.

In comparing the motor performances between boys and girls, in what general areas do boys out-perform girls and in what areas are girls superior to boys?

Girls tend to have better flexibility and balance than boys. Boys have broader shoulders and greater upper body strength. Those items requiring lower extremity strength and power are quite similar among boys and girls until the onset of adolescence, when boys make dramatic increasing while girls tend to follow a more linear increase.

What is the ideal and best method to assess biological maturity?

A skeletal examination (with x-rays), since its development spans the entire period of growth. These skeletal "bone age" films are usually taken of the wrist and compared to established x-rays in medical atlases (Greulich-Pyle Method). Three types of information regarding maturity may be gleaned from bone age x-rays. First, the appearance of specific bone centers which indicate the initial replacement of cartilage by bone tissue. Second is the definition of each bone by gradual shape differentiation as the adult form progressively becomes apparent. Third is the union or fusion of the epiphyses in the long bones of the radius, ulna, metacarpals and phalanges.

What differences are seen in leg length and sitting height during adolescence?

During the early adolescent growth spurt, the lower extremities grow faster than the upper extremities, giving the youngster the appearance of long legs. However, this disappears latter on during adolescence as the upper extremity catches up and thus, the sitting height increases.

❏❏ **What is the relationship between the development of peak strength and peak height velocity in males?**

In a study by Stolz and Stolz, more than 77% of the adolescent boys studied developed their peak strength after reaching their peak height velocity (PHV) whereas only 12% of the boys developed their peak strength before their PHV. Eleven percent of the male subjects developed their peak strength in concert with their PHV.

❏❏ **What is the relationship between the development of peak strength and peak height velocity in females?**

Unlike boys in the same study, more girls (40%) developed their peak strength before developing their peak height velocity (PHV). Forty-nine percent of the girls developed their peak strength after developing their PHV and 11% developed them concurrently.

❏❏ **How many fold(s) greater is (are) the peak strength gain (kg/ year) in boys versus girls?**

Twice. During their peak strength period, boys are able to perform an additional 12 kg per year while girls are able to perform an additional 6 kg per year.

❏❏ **In classifying a child for maturity status, what criterion is established for "normal" growth?**

Normal growth is established when the skeletal age is within plus or minus one year of the child's chronological age.

❏❏ **In terms of final stature, how do late maturers compare with early maturers?**

Late maturing adolescents eventually attain or perhaps surpass the stature of early maturing children.

❏❏ **How do final body proportions differ in early and late maturing children?**

Broader hips and narrower shoulders are characteristic of early maturing children. Late maturing children show the reverse, with broad shoulders and narrow hips. Leg length constitutes a greater percentage of height in late maturing children.

❏❏ **Which type of body morphology is associated with late maturation in males and females?**

Ectomorphy.

❏❏ **Describe the fat redistribution pattern in males during adolescence.**

Subcutaneous fat is lost on the extremities and redistributed more on the trunk.

❏❏ **Which type of body morphology is associated with early and advanced maturation in males?**

Mesomorphy.

❏❏ **Which type of body morphology is associated with early maturation in females?**

Endomorphy or a combination of endomorphy and mesomorphy.

❏❏ **At the conclusion of adolescence, how does maturity-associated variation factor into the overall strength in the male?**

Early maturing boys will be stronger at all ages than average and late maturing boys.

❏❏ **At the conclusion of adolescence, how does maturity-associated variation factor into the overall strength in the female?**

Early maturing females also show a similar pattern of increased strength compared to normal and late developing females. However, the difference is only marginal. As adolescence continues, this difference is reduced considerably.

❏❏ **How does the composition of water in the body change from the neonate to young adulthood periods?**

75% of the neonate's weight is attributed to water whereas only 62% of the young adult's weight is accounted for by water.

❏❏ **How does the composition of fat in the body change from the neonate to young adulthood periods?**

During the neonatal period, fat accounts for 15% of body weight for both sexes. In young adulthood, 25%- 30% of the female's weight is from fat whereas it only accounts for 12% to 16% of the male's weight.

❏❏ **Is regular exercise linked to increased stature?**

No. Contrary to the popular belief, studies show no apparent increase in height solely to regular exercising. Regular training results in a decrease in body fat, giving an appearance of increased height.

❏❏ **How does unilateral exercise (baseball pitching) affect the bones of the dominant arm?**

Radiographic studies show increased bone mineralization in the dominant arm when compared to the other arm.

❏❏ **Hypertrophy of which muscle type is associated with progressive strength training?**

Type II (fast-twitch) fibers.

❏❏ **Hypertrophy of which muscle type is associated with endurance training?**

Type I (slow-twitch) fibers.

❏❏ **What happens to the number of fat cells with regular exercise?**

Slimming down as a result of regular exercise is primarily from a reduction in fat cell size and not to changes in fat cell number.

❏❏ **Are there any ethnic group differences in terms of motor development?**

American Black children show a consistently marginal advanced motor development from infancy through 14.5 years of age compared to American White children. Differences between Mexican Americans and White infants were negligible.

❏❏ **Does the motor development of the first-born differ from his/her siblings?**

First-born children generally show more advanced motor behavior compared to his/her siblings. This, however, is usually related to greater maternal interaction and therefore stimulation of the first-born compared to later-born children.

❏❏ **What is the current thought on prepubescent strength training?**

Prepubescent boys can benefit from strength training contrary to previous belief. Studies on prepubescent girls are inconclusive.

❏❏ **How is the motor development different in families with opposite-sex siblings?**

Studies show that girls with older brothers tend to show more athletic interests than if they were to have older sisters. There have been no published studies on the motor development of boys with older sisters.

❏❏ **What values are set by the World Health Organization to be defined as hypertension in young adults?**

140/90 or higher.

❏❏ **By the time students graduate from high school, what percentage will be smokers?**

Almost 40%.

❏❏ **What is the correlation between excess body weight during infancy and latter life obesity?**

There is no correlation.

❏❏ **What is the relationship between menarche and exercising?**

Menarche is attained later in athletes than in non-athletes. There also seems to be a relationship between the delay in menarche and the more advanced competitive levels.

MEDICAL SCIENCE

EXERCISE PHYSIOLOGY

❑❑ As the height and mass of a person increases (within normal parameters), the amount of energy needed to perform a specific task increases or decreases?

Decreases through the concept of economy of running.

❑❑ What height-related feature can explain this phenomenon?

Stride length. Smaller people take shorter steps, taller people take longer steps (longer swing phase). The amount of energy used per step is similar, but more ground is covered by the larger person.

❑❑ Name the five components of physical fitness

Aerobic capacity, muscle flexibility, muscle strength, muscle endurance and body composition.

❑❑ Name the three energy-producing pathways or systems used by an athlete during physical activity.

Phosphocreatine (PC - burst energy), anaerobic (lactic acid), and aerobic.

❑❑ With each of the three energy systems, how many ATP units of energy are produced from a single molecule of glucose?

Aerobic system - 36 to 38 ATP units; Anaerobic system - 2 ATP units; Phosphocreatine system - 1 ATP unit.

❑❑ Approximately how long can an athlete doing maximal-effort work use the phosphocreatine (PC) energy system until exhausted?

Between 10 and 30 seconds.

❑❑ Approximately how long can an athlete perform work using the anaerobic energy system before reaching the anaerobic threshold?

Between one minute [minimally fit] and two minutes [well-conditioned]; and three minutes [world class athletes].

❑❑ **Name signs and symptoms demonstrated acutely upon reaching the anaerobic threshold.**

Elevated body temperature (begin to sweat), tachycardia, tachypnea, fatigue, burning in the muscles, muscle cramps.

❑❑ **What is the standard formula for approximating maximal heart rate?**

220 minus age.

❑❑ **When planning an aerobic workout, what is the range of percent of maximal heart rate that should be recommended as the target work zone?**

60 to 85%. Never exceed 85% of maximal heart rate for age for a sustained period of time. Such a workload is taxing to the cardiovascular system and could result in acute system failure (such as an acute myocardial infarction). Play it safe; at 85% of capacity, you will be working very hard, but your risk of a catastrophic event is quite small. Below 60%, you are giving an insufficient challenge to the cardiovascular system and aerobic energy system for the work being done. Boost up the workload to 60% and make more significant gains in fitness.

❑❑ **Below what percentage of relative workload (compared to maximal capacity) does the body recognize a given task as "easy, no sweat"?**

50%.

❑❑ **Above what percentage of relative workload does the body perceive a given task as very hard?**

85%.

❑❑ **What is the minimal length of time for an untrained person to achieve a minimally acceptable level of fitness in an exercise program?**

Three weeks.

❑❑ **What is the minimum number of days per week an individual must work out to maintain the level of fitness?**

Two.

❑❑ **What is the recommended number of days per week to engage in strength training for a given muscle group?**

Three to four days - alternating days on and days off. You can work out six days per week with strength training by doing upper body one day and lower body the next.

❑❑ **What is the recommended number of days per week to engage in stretching for flexibility by an individual engaged in a daily workout program?**

Daily - seven days per week; stretching daily.

❐❐ **The cardiac output for a young adult male increases by how many times during a moderate exercise program?**

Fourfold.

❐❐ **In designing a fitness program for a group such as a physical education class or an adult workout class, what is the weekly percentage of increased workload that can be handled by virtually every person with minimum risk of overuse injury?**

10% per week.

❐❐ **Using the 10% per week increase in workload guideline outlined above, how many weeks does it take to double one's workload?**

About seven weeks.

❐❐ **For a sedentary adult planning to make a lifelong commitment to fitness, what two words of wisdom are essential to understand in order to avoid overuse injuries?**

Gradualness and moderation. "Slow and Steady".

❐❐ **What is the term used to describe the utilization of a wide variety of physical activities for improving fitness?**

Cross training.

❐❐ **What method of stretching is considered to be better, ballistic (bouncing) or static?**

Static. Place the muscle on a stretch until you feel a gentle sense of pressure and tautness, but not pain. Hold each stretch for a minimum of 10 seconds, ideally for 30 seconds or more. Bouncing or ballistic stretches waste energy, stimulate stretch reflex receptors (causing the muscle you are trying to stretch to contract reflexively) and run the risk of tearing or straining the muscle.

❐❐ **If an athlete is focusing on improving flexibility as a prime goal of a fitness program, what is the time when the muscles will be most amenable to benefit from stretching?**

After a workout. The muscles are still warm and have been used in a manner which encourages them to be maximally pliant. Stretching at this time, being sure to hold each stretch for at least 30 seconds, will enable to the muscles to achieve new flexibility.

❐❐ **What is the reason why holding a static stretch for just over 30 seconds is considered ideal?**

The muscles are protected from rapid stretch by several inhibitory reflex organs. After these tendon reflex organs have been placed on a gentle stretch for more than 30 seconds, they temporarily defuse their sensitivity, allowing the muscle to stretch further without provoking an unconscious reflexive contraction of the particular muscle.

❑❑ What are several key principles and notions associated with strength training?

1. Overload principle - to get stronger, muscles must do more activity than they have done before; with small incremental increases, the body can respond to the challenge by improving.
2. Fatigue of the muscles is the goal; work muscles to exhaustion (the point of failure), but not to the point of pain or actual failure.
3. "No pain, no gain" is the wrong motto for "pumping iron" - pain indicates injury, not fitness.

❑❑ Resistance exercise has been shown to elevate human growth hormone (HGC) to what degree?

Anaerobic exercise (resistance strength training) - increases HCG levels 4 to 8 times
Aerobic exercise (moderate intensity, 30 minutes) - increases HCG levels 1 to 3 times.

❑❑ What is the range of repetitions generally recommended as safe and effective for an adult engaging in a strength training program using free weights?

The "7-11" rule or roughly similar guidelines are widely recommended for their efficacy and safety. Through trial and error, determine the weight at which one can accomplish a maximum of 7 repetitions until fatigue using the correct form for the exercise. Use this weight doing the training until such time as one can accomplish 11 such repetitions and still not be fatigued. At this point, repeat the process to find the new weight at which 7 repetitions can be accomplished. By using a weight that one can do seven repetitions, it is unlikely that one will be confronted with a situation which will cause injury.

❑❑ What are the general dangers in doing maximal lifts while strength training - or engaging in competitive weight lifting?

Since one is engaging in a maximal effort (1-RM or one repetition maximum), the possibility for failure is markedly heightened. If, for example, one was having an off day and was able to handle only 95% of the usual workload, confronting oneself with the full 100% workload might lead to immediate and complete failure on the part of the specific muscles. This is one of the reasons it is important to have spotters when bench pressing.

❑❑ What is the strength training zone? How does this relate to the relationship between number of repetitions to failure and percentage of 1 repetition maximum (1-RM)?

Since athletes engaging in strength training are discouraged from using a 1-RM, an appropriate zone for challenging muscles is needed. Activities that require less than 50% of 1-RM are not sufficiently challenging to produce significant gains unless the repetition number exceeds 30. Between 60% and 100% of the 1-RM, an essentially linear relationship exists between the number of repetitions to failure versus the load expressed as a percentage of 1-RM. At 60% of 1-RM, the number of repetitions to failure is between 15 and 20. The 7-11 relationship exists between 75% and 85% of 1-RM. In a fashion similar to how the aerobic target training zone is created, the strength training zone defines a safe yet effective window for improvement in fitness.

❑❑ **When engaging in a strength training program, how many sets of exercises are considered optimal?**

Three sets of repetitions to muscle fatigue (temporary failure) are considered optimal.

❑❑ **What is the technique of Progressive Resistance Exercise (PRE), devised after World War II by DeLorme?**

The DeLorme method of PRE involves three sets of exercises, each consisting of 10 repetitions done consecutively without rest. The first set involved one-half the maximum weight lifted ten times (or one-half 10-RM). The second set used three-quarters 10-RM; the final set required the full maximum weight for 10 repetitions, or 10-RM. As patients improved, their 10-RM resistance was adjusted periodically to match strength improvements. The basic DeLorme method continues to be used today with only minor modifications. The first set warms up the muscles (half of absolute maximum); the second set provides a challenge at 75% of maximum; the final set at the maximum provides the overload, being performed immediately after the warm-ups without intervening rest.

❑❑ **According to research using progressive resistance exercises (PRE), what are considered to be the range of the most effective number of repetitions to increase muscular strength?**

Research has determined that between 3-RM and 9-RM to fatigue is most effective. Since a 3-RM requires about 95% of 1-RM strength, it is not recommended for general populations because of the risk-benefit ratio. Under proper supervision in experienced athletes, 3-RM exercises can be appropriate for elite athletes.

❑❑ **Does weight training requiring heavy muscle contractions provide benefit for aerobic fitness (increase in VO_2max)?**

No significant improvement in aerobic capacity is demonstrated through strength training.

❑❑ **What is Delayed Onset Muscle Soreness (DOMS)?**

DOMS appears 24 hours after unaccustomed exercise and last as long as two weeks. Its effects are often most pronounced two to five days after activity. Cellular damage peaks during this time frame. Six factors are thought to be involved: (1) minute tears in muscle tissue, damaging cells, releasing chemical mediators that stimulate free nerve endings. (2) osmotic pressure changes cause fluid retention (swelling) in surrounding fibers. (3) muscle spasms or cramps (sudden, involuntary, severe contraction in a shortened position. (4) over-stretching and tearing of portions of the muscle's connective tissue harness (muscle-tendon junction). Microscopically, this is focused at the Z-line and involves myofibril damage. (5) alterations in the cell's mechanism for calcium regulation. (6) inflammation responses, causing increases in lymphocytes, interleukin-1 beta.

What type of muscle activity appears to cause more severe DOMS?

Eccentric muscle activity is associated with increased DOMS. High-force, high-tension eccentric muscle actions (actively resisting muscle lengthening) generally produce the greatest post-exercise damage and discomfort. This effect does not relate to lactate buildup because running (primarily concentric actions) produces no residual soreness despite significant elevations in blood lactate. In contrast, running downhill (primarily eccentric actions) causes moderate-to-severe DOMS without significantly elevation lactate during exercise.

What can be done to blunt or reduce DOMS?

Initiating an exercise program with a single bout of moderate concentric exercise provides a significant prophylactic effect on muscle soreness in subsequent high-force eccentric exercise with the effect persisting up to six weeks. Such results supports the wisdom of initiating a training program with repetitive, moderate concentric exercise to protect against muscle soreness that occurs following exercise with an eccentric component. Vitamin E, an antioxidant, thwarts free radical damage from lipid peroxidation. Vitamin E has been shown to reduce the effects of DOMS.

What is the danger of ingesting carbohydrates 30 minutes or less prior to exercise?

The combined effect of insulin release (responding to the elevated blood glucose level) and substrate utilization during exercise can lead to transient hypoglycemia, causing lightheadedness, fatigue and decreased performance.

Is there a danger of hypoglycemia if sugared fluids are ingested during exercise?

No. During high intensity exercise, the insulin effects are suppressed, allowing the blood sugar to be utilized (metabolized) during exercise.

Approximately how much fluid is carried within the cardiovascular system?

Systemic blood volume is five liters (about six quarts).

What is the volume of one pound of fluid?

Approximately one pint - sixteen ounces (actual amount is 453.6 grams or 16); two cups of fluid weigh about one pound.

When rehydrating oneself during exercise, is reliance on thirst a good indicator of fluid replacement requirement?

Thirst is a poor indicator of replacement fluid need. Individuals will under-drink if relying on thirst, taking in only about two-thirds of what is needed. By the time one's thirst mechanism kicks in, one can be 2% to 3% dehydrated. Athletes (and coaches) should schedule water breaks regularly throughout activity and athletes should consider drinking pre-determined specific amounts of fluid, rather than just quenching their thirst.

❑❑ **An active athlete is trying to maintain good hydration during activity. Create a drinking schedule during practice for fluid replenishment under usual summer conditions.**

Prior to starting activity, drink 13 to 20 ounces (400ml to 600ml) of fluid. Pre-exercise hyperhydration is helpful in preventing dehydration and heat illness. Drink 5 to 8 ounces of fluid every half-hour during activity; in extreme heat, it may be necessary to drink 5 to 8 ounces every 15 minutes. Try to have up to 15 minutes of rest or relative rest each hour. (McArdle/Katch/Katch, p.89)

❑❑ **Name the four standard ways the body loses water daily.**

In the urine, through the skin, as water vapor in expired air, and in feces.

❑❑ **What is the most significant health risk associated with acute weight reduction by an athlete during activity?**

Dehydration inducing heat illness. Heat illness has several grades and types, including heat cramps, heat fatigue, heat exhaustion and heat stroke.

❑❑ **What are the most commonly known signs of classical exertional heat stroke?**

Hot, dry skin and unconsciousness. The core temperature typically has risen to hyperthermic levels with the core temperature often at or above 106 degrees Fahrenheit. The body has become so depleted of circulating fluid that there is insufficient liquid to support circulation to the extremities and to produce sweat. Other common neurological signs of heat stroke include twitching, seizures, or marked disorientation as well as coma.

❑❑ **Name the four ways in which the body can dissipate heat and control core temperature.**

Conduction, convection, radiation and evaporation.

❑❑ **Describe how each of these methods can cool the core temperature. Discuss their limitations as well.**

Conduction is the process of heat being transferred to the surrounding medium. Air is a poor conductor and thus one does not dissipate body heat through conduction. Water, however, is an excellent conductor and readily transfers body heat; thus the cooling off in summer jumping into a swimming pool or lake. Metals are also good conductors and can absorb body heat. More commonly, however, the body relies on radiation and convection as heat loss mechanisms. *Radiation* heat loss (or gain) will occur when our un-insulated body is exposed to the ambient temperature. The difference between our core temperature (and skin temperature) and the air temperature will determine if heat is lost or gained. Stepping outside in winter without a coat will result in rapid heat loss through radiation into the cooler environment. By contrast, standing outside in the heat of the desert in summer (temperature well over 105 degrees Fahrenheit) will result in increasing our core temperature. *Convection* refers to the effects of air movement on heat loss. In still air, an athlete will radiate heat from his or her body, creating an envelope of warm air. As the athlete runs or the wind blows, that warmed pocket of air is moved away and replaced by air that can accept heat from the body. With significant speed of movement or wind speed, the cooling effect of the moving air becomes sufficiently significant that the term wind-chill factor becomes important. By far the most important method of cooling is *evaporation*, whereby sweat or water on our skin is absorbed into the air.

❑❑ How does evaporation cool our body and what are important considerations of this method of cooling?

Evaporation works by the state change of liquid water into gaseous water vapor, producing a cooling effect on the surface from where the water evaporated. One liter of sweat will release 600 kcal of heat energy from the body to the environment. Sweating *per se*, however, does not ensure cooling of the body. It is the evaporation, not the sweating, that causes the cooling effect. Further, it is not important if the water that evaporates came from sweat or sprinkling water on the surface of the skin; evaporation produces cooling. Any bead of sweat that falls to the ground or is wiped off with a towel is a bead of sweat that did not cool our body. In order for sweat to evaporate into the atmosphere, the air must be capable of absorbing the water vapor. Thus, if the relative humidity is approaching 100%, the atmosphere has essentially no interest in evaporating beads of sweat from active athletes, thus eliminating this important method of body cooling.

❑❑ What role does the ambient temperature have on temperature control during exercise?

When the environmental temperature is below 68 degrees, heat loss is mostly through convection and radiation from the skin. Above 68 degrees heat loss is through evaporative cooling.

❑❑ Explain why exercising during the heat of a summer's day could endanger an athlete's health.

When the air temperature is in the 90's (Fahrenheit) and the relative humidity is greater than 95% (and the wind speed is near zero), there are very limited ways to dissipate the heat generated by exercise. Radiation will not be effective since both the core temperature and air temperature are essentially equal. Convection will be of little benefit since the wind speed is negligible. Evaporation will be minimal since the air is already saturated with water vapor. One cannot effectively control the core temperature during exercise. Finally, the radiant heat caused by the powerful sun will raise core temperature even in the sedentary individual. Thus, strenuous exercise should be avoided; team practices should be canceled under such conditions.

❑❑ How long does it take for an athlete to become acclimatized to the heat?

Approximately four to ten days are needed to become accustomed to the heat. It is best to work out during the heat of the day, progressively doing a little more each day, to facilitate this process. An athlete is considered heat acclimatized when he can perform the required work (such as playing an entire game) while maintaining his body temperature within one degree centigrade (1.8 degrees Fahrenheit) of its normal range.

❏❏ **For a fit athlete who faces a hot environment for the first time, describe a logical plan to heat acclimatize over a four to ten-day period.**

Since the athlete is already fit from a cardiovascular, strength and endurance perspective, the goal here is simply to heat acclimatize. Working out in the heat on the first day, reduce the normal work out to 50% of usual. On each successive day, increase the amount of work done by 5% to 10%. Be sure to ingest plenty of fluids, electrolytes and other nutrients as needed.

❏❏ **What are some of the physiological adaptations the body uses to become heat acclimatized?**

The body increases its total body water by expanding blood volume. When exercise begins, the body begins to circulate blood to the extremities to enhance cooling through radiation and convection. The sweating mechanism is initiated sooner, producing sweat before the body temperature rises. The rate of sweat production also increases. The salt content of the sweat is more dilute than usual, thus preserving or minimizing salt loses through sweating.

❏❏ **For an athlete participating in a cross-country skiing race during winter in a cold, northern climate, what clothing considerations are important to help control body temperature?**

Dress in layers. When the race begins and the athlete is not generating large amounts of body heat, it is necessary to have multiple layers of clothing on to keep warm. As the race progresses and enormous quantities of heat are generated, it is necessary to shed layers of clothing to avoid overheating. The fabric polypropylene has the capacity to allow sweat to pass through it, allowing for cooling of the body through evaporation while still insulating the body from the cold surrounding environment. If the inner layers of clothing become and remain wet, they often lose their insulating capacity.

❏❏ **What is the most accurate method of monitoring the hydration status of an athlete?**

Athletes should weigh themselves, nude, before and after exercise.

❏❏ **When football teams begin fall practice during August, what important technique is used to monitor athletes during their heat acclimatization?**

Athletes are required to weigh in nude before and after each practice (especially during the two-a-day practice days). Athletes are required to rehydrate *to within two pounds of their initial weight on the first day* in order to be allowed onto the practice field for the next practice. As needed, trainers, athletes and coaches will develop a modified drinking plan to ensure weight maintenance within the required range.

❏❏ **What laboratory study can be useful in monitoring hydration status of an athlete?**

Urine color and urine specific gravity. When well hydrated, the urine of the athlete should be essentially clear and light in color; dehydrated athletes demonstrate dark, concentrated urine with a specific gravity above 1.020.

❏❏ **What is the minimum safe weight reduction endorsed by state high school associations for wrestlers on a weekly basis?**

Two to three pounds per week depending on the weight class.

❏❏ **How many calories can be generated from a pound of fat?**

3500 calories.

❏❏ **What is the recommended protein intake for an athlete trying to gain weight during resistance training?**

1.6 grams/kg of body weight or twice the RDA for protein for sedentary individuals.

❏❏ **What are some of the key principals of organizing a strength training prescription?**

Train the large core muscles first, then do the smaller stabilizing muscles. Train for power first, then for strength (rapid contraction movement for power first). Train the agonist and antagonist muscles during the same session (biceps and triceps, hamstrings and quads). Train muscles on alternate days (allowing time to consolidate muscular work into increased strength).

❏❏ **Which muscles and movements are included in the "core exercises"?**

The core exercises involve muscles that involve two or more joints and the large muscle groups. Power or quick lift exercises are those core exercises distinguishable by their ballistic nature and recruitment of "power zone" muscles (thighs to rib cage).

❏❏ **Provide several examples of core exercises, including power movement, quick lifts and other basic core exercises.**

Power movements-quick lifts: power snatch, power clean, hang snatch, hang clean, push press, push jerk, high pull (from floor and hang). Other core exercises: squat (front and back), quarter squat (front and back), leg press (hip sled), dead lift (with bent and straight legs), bench press, incline press, bent-over row, standing overhead press (in front and behind the neck).

❏❏ **What are the three basic principles of strength training?**

Overload (stimulus), adaptation (SAID principle - specific adaptation to imposed demands), and specificity (training in a specific manner to produce a specific outcome, such as strength, speed, endurance, power, etc).

❏❏ **When should athletes do strength training before practice and when should they do strength training after practice?**

During the pre-season and off-season, strength train first, then practice the sport. During the season, practice first, then strength train after practice. During the off-season and pre-season, gaining strength is the main goal; during the season, maintenance of strength is the key purpose.

❏❏ Describe the difference between an open kinetic chain exercise and a closed kinetic chain exercise?

Open chain kinetic exercises train a single muscle and have the distal end of the extremity "free and dangling", not bearing weight. While that single muscle gains in strength, there is no integrating of that muscle with its partners and neighbors. Closed kinetic chain exercises involve weight bearing through the distal end of the extremity, engaging not only the primary muscle to be trained, but the afferent nervous system sending proprioceptive information to higher levels. In addition, all of the muscles necessary for supporting that limb must contract as a team, at the proper moment and with the proper intensity to perform an activity in a smooth coordinated fashion.

❏❏ When performing lower extremity conditioning activities, which type of exercise is deemed more functional, open kinetic chain or closed kinetic chain?

Closed kinetic chain exercises are functional because they introduce the ground reactive forces of gravity and require the action of all muscles associated with an activity or action, not just a single muscle. Thus antagonist as well as agonist muscles are stimulated, as are muscles above and below the primary muscle being trained, and stabilizers as well as dynamic muscles are engaged. Open chain exercises concentrate on a single muscle.

❏❏ Name several responses of muscle to exercise.

(a) Muscle cells hypertrophy in size, (b) muscles improve motor control through repetitive exercise, (c) muscle cells improve by adaptive response of enzymes that decrease fatigue with sustained effort concurrently with (d) an increase in strength and (e) an increase in absolute endurance.

❏❏ Name the three common techniques (types of exercises) used in increasing muscle strength.

Isometric contraction (developing tension in the muscle although there is no movement of bones). An *isotonic* contraction (moving a fixed object or weight through the range of motion without regard to controlling speed); and an *isokinetic* contraction (moving through the range of motion at a fixed speed but without regard to the resistance from the object being moved).

❏❏ Is there scientific evidence for alternating days on and days off for strength training a given muscle group, or is this notion part of the "culture of training" without the benefit of scientific evidence?

There is scientific evidence for this notion. In a study on specificity of training at the University of Washington by DeLateur, two groups of individuals were trained in their quadriceps muscles using knee extensions, some at high resistance and few repetitions to achieve muscle fatigue and others at low resistance and high repetitions. After six weeks of training three times per week, they were tested using high resistance. As an incentive to perform their best, each person was offered money for each repetition they could do on *consecutive* days of testing. While the group that trained exactly as the testing protocol did better than those who trained using low resistance and high repetitions to fatigue, *NOT one single person* in the study could perform as many knee extensions the second day as they could the first day (even though they were being rewarded with money). This indicates that when muscles train to their maximum, they need time to recover and consolidate their gains in strength.

❏❏ **In weight lifting, what neural factors play a role in improved performance?**

"Learning" is often experienced during the first weeks of a strength training program. Learning represents the ability of the body to synchronize the firing of muscle fibers, thus contributing to a summation of forces. As time progresses and muscle hypertrophy, a single unit of electrical energy generates more total force because the larger muscle can produce more force when stimulated to contract.

❏❏ **If one limb is trained in a strengthening program, does the other untrained limb show any improvement in strength?**

Yes it does! There is no evidence for hypertrophy, but there is for improved isometric strength.

❏❏ **Name the two basic types of skeletal muscle fibers.**

Type I or slow twitch and Type II or fast twitch.

❏❏ **Fast twitch muscle fibers are associated with what types of activities and prefer which energy systems?**

Fast twitch fibers develop their tension rapidly. Fast twitch fibers are associated with explosive power generating activities and prefer the anaerobic energy systems (phosphocreatine system and anaerobic lactic acid system).

❏❏ **Slow twitch muscle fibers are associated with what types of activities and prefer which energy system?**

Slow twitch fibers develop tension more slowly. Slow twitch fibers are associated with endurance types of activities and preferentially use the aerobic energy system.

❏❏ **Under histological staining techniques, which fibers stain light and which stain dark?**

The type II (fast-twitch fibers) stain darkly.

❏❏ **Which muscle fibers reach fatigue more quickly?**

The fast-twitch Type II fibers, which use anaerobic metabolism, fatigue more quickly. There are two subtypes, Type IIa and Type IIb. Type IIb use primarily anaerobic glycolysis and fatigue rapidly; the Type IIa fibers are intermediate in reaching fatigue.

❑❑ **What role does the amount of glycogen stored in muscles play in the perceived exertion of an athlete doing a constant workload?**

If muscle glycogen stores are full, a given workload might be difficult but manageable. Repeating the identical work session when the muscle glycogen stores are below 25% at the start of the session, the athlete will experience significant fatigue and be unable to perform at the same level when done with full glycogen stores. With low muscle glycogen levels, the perceived exertion of a given activity is higher.

❑❑ **When is the body most receptive to reloading its glycogen stores following an exhaustive exercise session?**

Immediately after exercise, the body will most efficiently reload the muscle glycogen stores. By two hours after exercise, the rate of re-storage has declined, as it does by 8 hours and again by 24 hours. Thus athletes who will need to perform at a high level repeatedly (as in a tournament) should ingest a carbohydrate meal as soon after activity as possible.

❑❑ **Explain the difference between absolute workload and relative workload.**

Absolute workload indicates a set amount of work, such as lifting a 25-pound barbell. Relative workload is the proportion of the absolute workload to the capacity of that individual (a ratio). Assume that two people were asked to lift a 25-pound barbell, one whose maximum capacity was 50 pounds, and the other whose capacity was 200 pounds. The relative workload for the first individual would be 50% and the other would be 12.5% - even though both did exactly the same amount of work. For the person who relative workload was 50%, he or she would be working fairly hard to accomplish the task. For the person whose capacity was 200 pounds, this task qualifies for a "no sweat" comment.

❑❑ **Which is more important to muscle hypertrophy, intensity or duration of the workout?**

Intensity. A study by Mueller reported no muscle hypertrophy unless the intensity of the workout was at least 70% of the maximum contractile force.

❑❑ **During immobilization, when is muscle loss the greatest?**

The rate of muscle atrophy is greatest during the initial days of immobilization. After 5 to 7 days, the rate slows considerably.

❑❑ **How does the position of the limb during immobilization affect the amount of muscle atrophy?**

Muscles that are flexed or in a shorted position will atrophy more than muscles that are immobilized in an extended or stretched out position.

❑❑ **How are menstrual cramps typically managed for a female athlete?**

Excellent relief can be obtained by NSAIDs.

❐❐ **What are the mother's benefits of exercising during pregnancy?**

Weight control, improved muscle tone, self-esteem, decreased varicose veins, better sleep, decreased headache incidence, and a better sense of morale.

❐❐ **Obesity is defined as a body mass index (BMI) above what number?**

30.

❐❐ **What effect does exercise have on hypertension?**

After many literature reviews, a general consensus was reached in that exercise reduces resting blood pressure. It is estimated that the aerobic exercise reduces the systolic blood pressure by 5-25 mm Hg and the diastolic blood pressure by 3-15 mm Hg.

❐❐ **On the average, what percent of energy from ingested food is conserved for thermogenesis?**

10%.

❐❐ **The earliest sign of heat illness is generally heat cramps. Describe several key features of this condition.**

The combination of tightening muscle cramps and involuntary spasm of active muscles characterizes heat cramps. Low serum sodium levels are associated with heat cramps. Core temperature is still within normal limits.

❐❐ **Heat fatigue is another relatively early sign of heat illness. Describe several features of this condition.**

This condition is associated with decreased mental sharpness and ineffective performance and coordination. The athlete will feel somewhat lethargic as well. Movements will become awkward. Core temperature is still within normal limits.

❐❐ **Heat exhaustion is a serious form of heat illness. Describe its key features.**

As core temperature rises with exercise (up to 104°F or 40°C) and the body moves into significant negative water balance, the body recognizes imminent danger. Blood is pooling in the dilated peripheral vessels, dramatically reducing the central blood volume required to maintain adequate blood flow from the heart. The pulse is weak and rapid, blood pressure is low in the upright position, and headache, paleness, nausea, dizziness, "goose bumps" and general weakness are present. Sweating will be profuse initially and diminish as available body fluids decline even more.

❐❐ **If an athlete runs a marathon in over 3 hours, 30 minutes and drinks water as his only replacement fluid, what medical condition is he at risk for developing?**

Water intoxication. Consuming more than 9.5 liters can produce hyponatremia (when the serum sodium concentration falls below 136 mEq/liter. When the serum sodium falls below 130, symptoms such as headache, blurred vision, excessive sweating and vomiting appear. In extreme cases, patients many develop cerebral edema, becoming delirious, convulsive and comatose. This condition is more likely to afflict poorly conditioned individuals who perform high intensity exercise in hot weather and ingest frequent amounts of sodium-free fluid during their prolonged exercise (such as someone's first marathon). Well-conditioned athletes can also be at risk in such activities as ultramarathons and the Ironman Triathlon, where 6 to 8 hours of high-intensity, continuous exercise can stress the body's physiologic systems.

☐☐ **For athletes doing strenuous exercise of one hour or less, what is the recommended fluid for rehydration?**

Water is preferred for fluid replacement for activities under 90 minutes in length. After that length of time, electrolyte losses become more significant and electrolyte containing drinks are indicated.

☐☐ **To assist in rehydration during activity, what is the preferred temperature for replacement fluids?**

Cold fluids (41°F, 5°C) empty the stomach at a faster rate than fluids at body temperature.

☐☐ **If using sweetened electrolyte-containing fluids, what considerations for percentage of carbohydrate and osmolarity are needed?**

Gastric emptying slows down when the ingested fluid contains concentrated electrolytes or simple sugars. For example, a 40% sugar solution empties at a rate 20% slower than plain water. As a general rule, between a 5% or 8% carbohydrate-electrolyte beverage consumed during exercise in the heat contributes to temperature regulation and fluid balance as effectively as plain water. As an added bonus, this drink helps maintain glucose metabolism and glycogen reserves in prolonged exercise.

☐☐ **In regard to fluid rehydration during exercise, what six physiological factors affect gastric emptying?**

In general, (1) increased volume increases the emptying rate; (2) increased caloric content decreases the emptying rate; (3) increased solute concentration (osmolarity) decreases emptying rate; (4) exercise intensity exceeding 75% of maximum decreases emptying rate; (5) marked deviations from a pH of 7.0 decrease emptying rate; and (6) dehydration decreases gastric emptying and increases risk of gastrointestinal distress.

☐☐ **In regard to fluid rehydration during exercise, what three physiological factors affect intestinal fluid absorption?**

Low to moderate levels of glucose plus sodium increases fluid absorption. Low to moderate levels of sodium increase fluid absorption. Hypotonic-to-isotonic fluids containing NaCl and glucose increase fluid absorption.

☐☐ **Within each muscle sarcomere, describe the geometric relationship of actin and myosin filaments.**

The thick myosin myofilaments are surrounded by six actin myofilaments in a hexagonal array. Each actin filament contributes to three myosin filaments. Myosin filaments produce spiral crossbridges that reach out and can both attach to the actin and rotate in space (creating a sliding filament action). One end of the actin filament is secured to the "z-line" of the sarcomere.

❏❏ Explain how myosin and actin myofilaments mechanically move in relation to each other.

Myosin crossbridges are spiral projections around the myosin filaments with globular, lollipop-like head which extend perpendicularly and interact with the actin filaments. Tropomyosin and troponin, the two most important constituents of the actin helix structure, regulate the make-and-break contacts between myofilaments during muscle action. Tropomyosin inhibits actin and myosin coupling and prevents permanent bonding. Troponin (in conjunction with the calcium ion) triggers myofibrils to interact and slide past each other. The globular head of the myosin forms an actinomyosin crossbridge. This arrangement provides the mechanical power stroke for actin and myosin filaments to slide past each other. These actions resemble that of oars in the water moving a crew shell. But unlike the crew team, the crossbridges do not all move synchronously. More specifically, after forming the actinomyosin crossbridge, the elongated flexible myosin globular head literally bends around the ATP molecule and becomes cocked like a spring. The myosin then interacts with the ATP, producing a sliding motion that initiates muscle shortening as it breaks the actinomyosin crossbridge.

❏❏ How do calcium ions facilitate muscle contraction?

In the relaxed state, where few calcium ions are present, troponin and tropomyosin interact and prevent actin and myosin binding. When the muscle contracts, calcium ions the sarcomere enter from the lateral vesicles of the sarcoplasmic reticulum; the calcium binds to a binding site on the troponin, releasing the inhibitory effect of the tropomyosin. The myosin globular head now creates a crossbridge of actinomyosin, developing tension. ATP is necessary to help release the actin-myosin crossbridge regenerating actin and myosin. The energy generated during the release of the actinomyosin crossbridge creates the classic movement of the filaments to move past one another. Once the level of calcium ions drops to baseline levels, muscle contraction chemistry is restored to the resting state. This is achieved through active transport pumps.

❏❏ Explain the terms eccentric and concentric contractions.

When muscles develop tension, chemical bonds are formed between the actin and myosin molecules. If tension develops and no movement takes place, the term isometric is applied. Most commonly, muscles develop tension while shortening in length. The combination of developing tension while shortening is termed a concentric contraction. There are times, however, when muscle must develop tension while lengthening. In such case, development of tension as a muscle lengthens is called an eccentric contraction. This often occurs when an agonist-antagonist force couple work as a team. Two examples of eccentric contraction include doing a controlled slow elbow extension with a dumbbell weight against gravity; and when the quadriceps forcibly contracts to extend the knee, the hamstrings engage eccentrically to prevent hyperextension of the knee, providing a braking action to the leg.

❑❑ What is plyometric muscle training?

Plyometric training makes use of the inherent stretch-recoil characteristics of skeletal muscle and neurological modulation via the stretch or myotactic reflex. Their goal is to develop speed strength. The stretch shortening cycle describes the linked muscle actions of eccentric-isometric-concentric contractions seen in such activities as walking and jumping. When stretching occurs rapidly, stored elastic energy in muscle fibers and the initiation of the myotactic reflex combine to produce a powerful concentric contraction. Faster recruitment of muscle fibers and recruitment of more muscle fibers with prior stretching may also augment a muscle's response. Two examples include depth jumping and reactive ability (jumping from boxes).

❑❑ What are several key safety issues associated with plyometric training?

Because of the explosive nature of plyometric training, a baseline level of strength relative to body weight is necessary to perform these exercises safely and effectively. Plyometrics should be done no more frequently than one to three times per week. Plyometrics should not be performed on the same body area on days when heavy resistance exercises or other intense activities are scheduled. Wait at least 48 hours to allow for recovery before repeating plyometrics on a given body area.

❑❑ With plyometric training, what are the general guidelines for number of foot or hand contacts per session?

Beginner should limit themselves to 80 to 100 total contacts, intermediates between 100 to 120, and advanced between 120 and 140 total contacts of hands or feet.

❑❑ Compare the concentration of electrolytes in the serum and in sweat.

Sweat has less sodium than serum, making it hypotonic (lower osmolarity) compared to serum. Specifically, blood serum has a sodium concentration of approximately 140meq/l, sweat has 40-45; potassium: serum 4.0; sweat 3.9; chloride: serum 110; sweat 39; magnesium: serum 1.5-2.1, sweat 3.5. As the body acclimatizes, the plasma blood volume rises and sweat production increases. The electrolyte content of sweat decreases, permitting the body to conserve electrolytes.

❑❑ What is the caloric energy derived from the metabolism of one gram of carbohydrate, protein and fat?

Carbohydrate and protein generate 4 calories/gram while fat generates 9 calories/gram.

❑❑ What in interval training and why is it beneficial?

Interval training entails interspersing periods of intense physical exercise within an exercise regimen. Between intervals, there is a recovery period, which may be exercise at a lower level of activity. This type of aerobic training usually lasts three to five minutes when the athlete trains at speeds above racing speed. The recovery period is generally one to one-and-one-half times the length of the interval and is at a level between 30% and 50% of VO_2max. The number of intervals is inversely related to their length; shorter intervals (3 minutes) should be repeated 5 to 10 times per session; longer intervals (5 minutes) may be repeated 4 to 5 times per session. Because of the specificity of running as the modality, interval training is especially effective for distance runners.

❑❑ **In what ways can interval training be detrimental to the athlete?**

Because of the extra challenges associated with interval training, running for several minutes at a faster pace than racing speed, the amount of force the legs must dissipate increases, raising the risk of overuse injuries.

MEDICAL SCIENCE

PHARMACOTHERAPEUTICS

❑❑ **Name four techniques that are useful in the exercising diabetic athlete that prevent adverse effects of vigorous exercise on blood glucose.**

Prior to exercise do not inject insulin in a muscle site that will be heavily used in the competition or practice. Monitor blood glucose closely before, during and for 24 hours after vigorous exercise. Delay or reduce vigorous exercise if blood glucose is not in the 100 - 250 mg/dl range. Reduce dosage of insulin by 30 - 50 % depending on intensity of exercise, duration of event and prior experience with vigorous exercise.

❑❑ **In an asthmatic athlete who is experiencing acute bronchospasm, what is the drug of choice?**

A short acting *B* agonist such as albuterol is effective for rescue therapy in an asthmatic athlete.

❑❑ **In an athlete with a history of exercise induced bronchospasm how would you recommend using a short acting bronchodilator for prophylaxis?**

Albuterol may be given 15 - 30 minutes prior to practice or a competitive event.

❑❑ **T/F: Leukotriene modifiers such as Montelukast have be shown to be effective in the treatment of exercise induced bronchospasm.**

True. Although these agents are not regarded as first line medications, they have been shown to be effective in controlling exercise induced bronchospasm in asthmatics with persistent asthma.

❑❑ **T/F: Epinephrine injections are the drug of choice for the prevention of exercise induced anaphylaxis.**

False. Parenteral epinephrine is the drug of choice in the treatment of exercise induced anaphylaxis once it has developed. Non sedating antihistamines are the drugs of choice for the prevention of this condition.

❑❑ **Which category of antibiotics are associated with an increased risk of tendon rupture?**

Fluoroquinolones.

❑❑ **Which enzyme in the production of prostaglandins is inhibited by non steroidal anti inflammatory drugs and salicylates?**

NSAIDs and salicylates inhibit cycle oxygenase, the enzyme that converts arachidonic acid to the prostaglandins.

❑❑ **Which enzyme in the inflammatory process is inhibited by corticosteroids?**

Corticosteroids reduce the production of arachidonic acid by inhibiting phospholipase.

❑❑ **Which category of antihypertensive medications is least likely to adversely affect athletic performance?**

ACE inhibitors.

❑❑ **In addition to the tetracyclines, which other medications are known to have phototoxic reactions in athletes who are exposed to bright sunlight?**

Griseofulvin, chlorothiazide, chlorpropamide, sulfa antibiotics and chlordiazepoxide.

❑❑ **Which diuretic is useful in managing athletes who are susceptible to acute mountain sickness?**

Acetazolamide starting 24 hours prior to ascent to altitudes greater than 2400 meters (8000 feet) reduces the signs and symptoms of acute mountain sickness.

❑❑ **What physiologic parameters are altered by acetazolamide?**

Acetazolamide inhibits the enzyme carbonic anhydrase. CO_2 production and retention are reduced. These parameters, plus possible additional effects of acetazolamide on cerebrospinal fluid production, decrease the signs and symptoms of acute mountain sickness.

❑❑ **T/F: Topical antibiotics are effective in the treatment of swimmer's ear (otitis externa)**

True. Otitis externa is treated with topical antibiotics which include neomycin and polymyxin B. Systemic antibiotic are usually unnecessary.

❑❑ **What is the treatment of choice for Tinea pedis (athlete's feet)?**

Topical antifungal medications such as clotrimazole, miconazole or econazole.

❑❑ **T/F: Patients with widespread fungal infections (tinea corporis) should be treated with systemic antifungals such as griseofulvin.**

True.

❏❏ **T/F: Systemic steroids have been shown to be effective in reducing the pain and inflammation of sunburn.**

False. Systemic steroids have been evaluated and found to be no better that placebo in the treatment of pain and inflammation related to sunburn.

❏❏ **What is the most commonly used drug in the management of increased intracranial pressure in aduts?**

Mannitol. It is used commonly as a 20 % solution, initially given as a bolus of 1 g/kg IV bolus. Since it can aggravate hypovolemia, it should not be given to a hypotensive patient.

❏❏ **T/F: Hypotension is often associated with the use of barbiturates in the management of increased intracranial pressure. Therefore, they are not recommended in the head injured athlete who is hypotensive.**

True.

❏❏ **List some of the side effects of antihistamines used in the treatment of allergic rhinitis which can be detrimental to athletic performance.**

Drowsiness.
Lethargy.
Dry mucous membranes.
Nausea.
Lightheadedness.

❏❏ **Nonsteroidal anti-inflammatory agents (NSAIDs) are often used because of their analgesic and anti-inflammatory properties in the management of bruises, strains and sprains. When used on a continuous basis for more than 4-5 days up to 50% of patients will experience side effects. What type of side effects would you anticipate?**

Abdominal pain.
Dyspepsia.
Heartburn.
Nausea.

❏❏ **What effect do corticosteroids have on wound healing?**

They have been associated with the arrest of the inflammatory phase of wound healing.

❏❏ **What side effects are associated with the use of angiotensin converting enzyme (ACE) inhibitors used in the treatment of the hypertensive athlete?**

Cough. Hyperkalemia can occur when these drugs are used in combination with nonsteroidal anti-inflammatory agents.

❏❏ **T/F: Hydrochlorothiazide can be associated with dehydration in athletes.**

True.

❏❏ **Which two injection sites should be avoided when administering injectable steroids because of their propensity to rupture?**

Patellar tendon.
Achilles tendon.

❏❏ **Identify three potential dermatological complications of corticosteroids.**

Hypopigmentation.
Hyperpigmentation.
Subcutaneous atrophy.

❏❏ **When is the peak activity of regular insulin?**

Two to four hours.

❏❏ **What recommendation would you make to the diabetic athlete with regard to the anticipated peak insulin activity?**

Do not exercise at the time of peak insulin action.

❏❏ **What effect does exercise have on the absorption of human and porcine insulin?**

Both are absorbed faster with exercise; porcine slightly more.

❏❏ **What is the drug of choice for treating the athlete with primary syphilis?**

Benzathine penicillin G.

❏❏ **Trichomonas vaginalis is the most common cause of sexually transmitted vaginitis. What treatment regimen would you suggest to the athlete whose wet mount preparation showed motile trichomonads and whose clinical signs and symptoms were consistent with this infection?**

Metronidazole: 2g PO, single dose or 250 mg PO tid x 7 days.

❏❏ **Why is an allergic athlete who is using alpha adrenergic agents (decongestants) at increased risk for heat emergencies?**

These agents are associated with vasoconstriction and limited blood flow to the skin.

❏❏ **T/F: Salt tablets are recommended in the management of heat cramps.**

False. Salt tablets are not indicated because of their irritant effect on the gastrointestinal tract.

❏❏ **A swimmer presents with ear pain. The external auditory canal is erythematous and swollen. A watery discharge is noted and pain is elicited with manipulation of the auricle. The tympanic membrane appears normal. How would you treat this patient?**

This scenario is consistent with a diagnosis of external otitis. The external canal should be cleansed and antibiotic eardrops with or without steroids and / or drying agent should be recommended.

❏❏ **Acetazolamide has been used in the treatment of mild Acute Mountain sickness. What are some of the adverse effects that can be seen with this drug?**

Peripheral paresthesias, polyuria.
Less commonly nausea, drowsiness.
Taste perversion.

❏❏ **Under what circumstances might you recommend acetazolamide?**

Rapid ascent to altitude over 3000 meters.
History of recurrent Acute Mountain sickness or high altitude pulmonary edema.
Treatment of Acute mountain sickness.
Periodic breathing or fragmented disturbed sleep at altitude.

❏❏ **What is a steroid flare?**

Steroid flare is a term that refers to pain at the site of the steroid injection. It is caused by the precipitation of crystals.

❏❏ **Oral contraceptives are frequently used by female athletes to prevent unwanted pregnancies. What are some of the side effects you should discuss that may impact on their sports performance?**

Dizziness, migraine headaches, lethargy, hypertension, urinary tract infections and dysmenorrhea.

❏❏ **Which injectable medication is associated with muscle atrophy that may be permanent?**

Anti-inflammatory steroids.

❏❏ **Which infectious disease, that is considered a pre-emptive condition for wrestling is treated with antiviral medications?**

Herpes gladiatorum.

❏❏ **T/F: Inhaled steroids that are used as a maintenance medication to control asthma in an athlete are banned substances in elite Olympic levels of competition.**

False.

❏❏ **T/F: Oral Albuterol that is used to control an acute exacerbation of asthma in an elite Olympic athlete is not permitted during competition.**

True.

❏❏ **T/F: Albuterol delivered by metered dose inhaler (MDI) to treat an acute exacerbation of asthma in an elite Olympic athlete is always permitted during competition.**

False. Albuterol MDI is only permitted during competition at Olympic events if the athlete and the athlete's pulmonologist or team physician has notified the national governing body or the doping control authority of the use of these products prior to competition.

MEDICAL SCIENCE

ERGOGENIC AIDS

❏❏ **Anabolic-androgenic steroids have a positive effect on which of the following components of exercise physiology?**

Muscle strength and muscle mass.

❏❏ **The dietary supplement Creatine is in which biochemical category?**

A nucleic acid.

❏❏ **Higher doses of caffeine resulting in urinary levels greater than 12mcg/mL are more likely to positively enhance sports performance in competition lasting what length of time?**

30 minutes to 60 minutes.

❏❏ **What is Guarana?**

Guarana is a stimulant produced from a Brazilian herb and contains multiple substances the most significant of which is caffeine (2.5%-5% by weight).

❏❏ **Dietary supplements are regulated by which federal agency?**

FDA (food and drug administration).

❏❏ **Dietary supplements are regulated under which legislative mandate?**

Dietary supplement health and education act 1994.

❏❏ **Do either the FDA and the DEA routinely test dietary supplements for content, consistency or quality?**

No, not until a complaint is filed with the specific agency.

❏❏ **The term "stacking" is used by individuals who abuse ergogenic drugs to describe which technique?**

The use of multiple drugs in a regimen intended to maximize desired effects, minimize negative side effects, and/or avoid detection in drug testing scenarios.

❐❐ **The term "cycling" is used by individuals who abuse ergogenic drugs to describe which technique?**

The use of multiple drugs in a sequence to maximize desired effects, minimize negative side effects, and/or avoid detection in drug testing scenarios.

❐❐ **Do Anabolic steroid precursors such as androstenediol, androstenedione, and dehydroepiandrosterone affect serum testosterone levels in individuals who use these products?**

Use of these drugs results in brief (1-2 hour) elevations in serum testosterone levels.

❐❐ **Are dietary supplements such as androstenediol, androstenedione, and dehydroepiandrosterone banned in elite Olympic competition?**

Yes, these products can result in a positive test for anabolic steroids.

❐❐ **Are cholestatic jaundice and hepatic transaminase elevations that result from use and abuse of anabolic-androgenic reversible?**

Yes, these parameters commonly revert to baseline following cessation of use of these drugs making measurement of bilirubin and transaminase levels of limited use in detecting use of these products.

❐❐ **Do anabolic-androgenic steroids cause testicular cancer?**

Although concern has been voiced in the popular literature, there has not been a scientific link established between anabolic-androgenic steroid use and the risk of testicular cancer in young male athletes.

❐❐ **Do anabolic-androgenic steroids cause hypertrophic cardiomyopathy?**

Although in vitro studies have prompted concern regarding the risk of hypertrophic cardiomyopathy and the use of anabolic-androgenic steroids, the correlation between these has not been established conclusively in the clinical literature.

❐❐ **Do anabolic-androgenic steroids increase the risk of myocardial infarct?**

Anabolic-androgenic drug use is a risk factor in the development of atherosclerotic heart disease in that these drugs adversely affect lipid profiles and the risk of hypertension.

❐❐ **Do dietary supplements such as androstenediol, androstenedione, and dehydroepiandrosterone increase the risk of male pattern baldness?**

These dietary supplements, with prolonged use, have the same effects and the same side effects as other anabolic-androgenic steroids including their adverse effects on the integumentary system.

❑❑ **T/F: Linear height growth arrest is a side effect of anabolic androgenic steroids in all athletes who use and abuse these products.**

False Linear height growth arrest is a side effect of anabolic-androgenic only in skeletally immature young athletes due to premature closure of the epiphyseal growth plate secondary to accelerated pubertal development.

❑❑ **T/F: Nicotine containing products, including chewing gum, oral snuff, cigarettes, and dermal patches may result in mild stimulation during athletic event.**

True, however the degree of performance enhancement in small. Cigarettes and smokeless tobacco products are prohibited by many sports governing bodies because of adverse effects on the athlete's health.

❑❑ **T/F: Ephedrine is a stimulant derived from plants in the genus Ephedra and is a banned stimulant.**

True. Even though this chemical is currently a loosely regulated dietary supplement, it has significant performance enhancement characteristics and is a prohibited substance at collegiate and Olympic competition. Related substances contained in herbal teas, products such as gingko biloba, and ginseng are also prohibited and tested for.

❑❑ **What are the ergogenic benefits of ephedrine in athletic competition?**

Decreased perception of fatigue, increased mental alertness. These positive effects are offset by adverse effects on coordination, hydration, and thermoregulation.

❑❑ **Is PPA (phenylpropanolamine) a banned stimulant at elite levels of competition?**

This metabolic stimulant has a positive ergogenic effect on performance and is banned in the stimulant category. The active ingredient in many decongestant product and dietary aids, it has recently been removed from the market because of an increase risk of hemorrhagic stroke in women 19-49 who were using this product in over the counter dietary products.

❑❑ **Are stimulant controlled substances (amphetamine derivatives and methylphenidate) that are used for management of attention disorders in children and adults prohibited substances?**

These products have significant ergogenic effects on performance and are banned at elite levels of competition.

❑❑ **What is "Khat"?**

Athletes may disclose to their primary care physician that they are including Khat in their dietary regimen. Khat is a herbal product derived from Catha edulis and contains cathine and cathinone which are amphetamine-like stimulants. Products containing these chemicals are banned substances at the elite level of competition.

❑❑ **Is Echinacea a banned or prohibited substance in athletic competition?**

Echinacea is a herbal medication derived from a plant that is native to the American prairie, the cone-flower. In its pure form it has not been shown to have an ergogenic effect and, as such, is not a banned substance in most areas of competition. Difficulties with manufacturing and adulteration of these products with other substances that are banned has caused an almost universal warning to elite athletes that they take products containing echinacea at their own risk.

❑❑ **Name four physiologic parameters that increase the risk of stroke from hyperviscosity syndrome.**

1. Congenital conditions predisposing an individual athlete to hypercoagulation.
2. High osmotic diet load secondary to the use of dietary supplements.
3. Dehydration.
4. Hematocrit elevation beyond 55% secondary to EPO or autologous blood transfusion.

❑❑ **T/F: Plasma expanders, such as hetastarch, are used by athletes to enhance performance in brief, explosive power sports.**

False, these products are most commonly seen in athletes competing in endurance events and are banned substances at elite levels of competition.

❑❑ **T/F: Autologous blood transfusions, similar to EPO, may result in hematocrits above 65%.**

False. Packed cell transfusion results in hematocrits in the range of 50-55%.

❑❑ **Human growth hormone (HGH) is used by athletes to enhance which physiologic parameters?**

Enhance linear growth in skeletally immature athletes (no effect on linear growth on skeletally mature athletes), increase body weight, increase muscle mass, however the effect of HGH on muscle strength is limited

❑❑ **T/F: Supplemental HGH use results in clinical acromegaly in skeletally mature athletes.**

True.

❑❑ **How does Human Chorionic gonadotropin (hCG) enhance body weight and increase muscle mass in athletes?**

These effects are produced in the human body by hCG's effect on endogenous testosterone production secondary to its stimulation of testosterone production by the adrenal glands and the testes.

❏❏ **Propranolol and other beta-blockers are used by athletes to alter which performance parameters?**

Athletes use these products to lower heart rate in sports (archery and shooting) where fine motor tremulousness is detrimental to performance and to increase the endogenous production of human growth hormone.

❏❏ **T/F: Beta-agonists such as albuterol are prohibited substances at elite levels of competition.**

False. Oral and parenteral preparations of these products are prohibited. Inhaled forms of these products are "restricted" in athletes who use these products to treat reactive airway disease. They are required to notify, in advance, their sport's governing body. At the Olympic level the diagnosis of asthma must be made or confirmed by a pulmonologist/ allergist or the team physician.

❏❏ **Diuretics such as furosemide are used by athletes in attempts to alter which competitive parameters?**

Athletes use these products to mask the use of other illicit ergogenic drugs in drug testing scenarios, to reduce the water retention side effects of other ergogenic drugs, and to reduce body weight in weight category dependent competition.

❏❏ **T/F: Alcohol (ethanol) is an ergogenic aid.**

True. It has limited use as a source of energy substrates and is a potential adverse ergogenic product because of adverse effects on muscle coordination, mental alertness, and muscle endurance due to dehydrating effects. It is a banned substance in sports where reduction of heart rate and fine motor tremulousness is a competitive advantage.

❏❏ **T/F: Chromium is a mineral used by athletes to enhance muscle metabolism.**

True. However, the effectiveness of chromium on muscle metabolism in competitive scenarios is questionable. Chromium is often taken as chromium picolinate to enhance oral absorption. Athletes are aware that chromium is a co-factor for insulin. However, there is limited and often contradictory data on whether supplementation of this mineral is ergogenic.

❏❏ **T/F: Supplementation of sodium bicarbonate is useful as an ergogenic aid by reducing lactic acidosis during competition.**

False. The amounts of sodium bicarbonate that would be required to significantly affect lactic acid metabolism at the muscle tissue level would be so large that the sodium load and water requirements would likely result in significant performance reduction.

❏❏ **T/F: Tribulus is effective in increasing endogenous testosterone production.**

False. Tribulus is a derivative of an oriental plant (tribulus terrester). Young athletes use this product because it is marketed for its effect on testosterone production. It has not been shown to significantly increase testosterone production either when used alone or in combination with other products. It has not been shown to enhance performance in competitive scenarios.

❑❑ **T/F: Clenbuterol, an inhaled beta agonist, is a banned substance because of its anabolic effect on muscle tissue.**

True.

❑❑ **T/F: Use of alcohol increases the risk of nitrogen narcosis during SCUBA diving.**

True. An increased risk of injury in SCUBA diving is also seen because of poor judgment and spatial disorientation in divers who ingest alcohol.

❑❑ **Which amino acid has been shown to increase endurance in swimmers?**

Choline.

❑❑ **Why do athletes supplement their diets with branched chain amino acids such as isoleucine, leucine and valine?**

Athletes add additional branched chain amino acids to the diet in attempts to increase the amount of tryptophan in their system and consequently alter perception of muscle fatigue.

❑❑ **Which amino acid is used by athletes to improve efficiency of fatty acid metabolism?**

L-carnitine.

❑❑ **What physiologic parameters are athletes trying to enhance by supplementing their diets with cyanocobalamin (Vitamin B-12)?**

Increased RBC production and possibly enhanced nerve / muscle efficiency.

❑❑ **Which parameters are athletes attempting to alter by using products that contain vanadium, a trace mineral?**

Vanadium, vanadyl sulfate, and related products are used for their purported insulin-like effects. Although increased transport of glucose was noted in laboratory animals, there is limited data available as to the effect, lack of effect, or potential side effects of these products.

❑❑ **Which physiological parameters are affected by dietary supplementation with Beta-hydroxy-beta-methylbutyrate?**

Beta-hydroxy-beta-methylbutyrate (HMB) is used by athletes in attempts to increase muscle strength and lean body mass. This compound is a metabolite of the amino acid leucine.

❏❏ **Why do athletes supplement their diet with Glutamine?**

Glutamine, a non-essential amino acid, has been studied in athletes in order to determine whether it counters the adverse effect that vigorous training has on an athlete's immune system.

❏❏ **What effect does Coenzyme Q-10 have on exercise physiology parameters?**

CoenzymeQ-10 (ubiquinone) facilitates aerobic generation of ATP and functions as an antioxidant. The degree to which Coenzyme Q-10 supplementation enhances athletic performance is equivocal.

❏❏ **Which parameters are athletes who supplement their diets with products that contain chemicals referred to as "oryzanols" attempting to enhance?**

Plant sterols that are referred to as "oryzanols" are related to ferulic acid, a compound that athletes use for its purported antioxidant effects and for its possible effects on growth hormone secretion.

MEDICAL SCIENCE

NUTRITION

❑❑ **Does carbohydrate ingestion improve athletes performance during endurance events?**

Only during endurance events lasting > 1 hour.

❑❑ **What is the carbohydrate recommendation during training for endurance athletes?**

30 – 60 g/hr of carbohydrate rich foods or fluids.

❑❑ **What is the carbohydrate recommendation following prolonged exercise?**

1.5 g/kg within 30 minutes of exercise and an additional 1.5 g/kg within 2 hours.

❑❑ **T/F: The average American diet provides excess fat for sedentary people but adequate amounts for athletes.**

False. The average American diet has too much fat for both athletes and non athletes alike.

❑❑ **Overnight fasts are not recommended for athletes. Why?**

Overnight fasts are associated with lowered liver glycogen stores which can cause hypoglycemia and fatigue.

❑❑ **Are there any advantages to liquid over solid meals prior to exercise?**

Liquid meals are associated with more rapid gastric emptying times. This may help to prevent nausea.

❑❑ **T/F: Runner's anemia can occur as a transient phenomenon during the early stages of strenuous physical training, especially among female athletes.**

True.

❑❑ **What is water's most important function in the athlete?**

Regulation of body temperature.

❐❐ **What is the most appropriate replacement fluid for exercise lasting ≤ 1 hour?**

Water.

❐❐ **Why are athletes advised to avoid carbonated beverages prior to exercise?**

They may cause gastrointestinal discomfort.

❐❐ **What is the major source of electrolyte loss during exercise?**

Sweat.

❐❐ **What is the electrolyte concentration of human sweat?**

Each liter of sweat contains about 10 to 30 mEq of sodium and 3 to 10 mEq of potassium.

❐❐ **T/F: In conditioned and acclimated athletes, sweating usually does not cause electrolyte imbalance.**

True.

❐❐ **T/F: In unacclimated athletes exposed to extreme conditions and /or heavy fluid losses electrolyte imbalances can occur.**

True.

❐❐ **T/F: Vitamin supplements have been shown to improve athletic performance.**

False. Studies have not shown improved performance in athletes taking vitamin supplements over those taking placebo.

❐❐ **What are the benefits of exercise in weight loss programs?**

Promoting fat loss while maintaining lean body mass.
Promoting healthy lifestyle.

❐❐ **What dietary recommendations would you make to an athlete with runner's diarrhea?**

Eat a low fiber diet 24 to 36 hours prior to competition.
Eliminate foods that trigger bowel irritation, including lactose, if athlete is intolerant.
Improve hydration before and during exercise.

❐❐ **T/F: Carbohydrates, fats and proteins make up the macronutrients that ultimately provide the energy necessary to maintain bodily functions during activity.**

True.

❏❏ **Which macronutrient serves as the most significant fuel source during high intensity exercise?**

Carbohydrates primarily serve as the energy fuel, particularly during high intensity exercise.

❏❏ **T/F: Many studies have demonstrated that carbohydrate supplementation increases endurance.**

True.

❏❏ **T/F: Cholesterol is the most widely known lipid. Although it may be found in both plants and animals, the majority of it exists in animal tissue.**

False. Cholesterol is only found in animal tissue.

❏❏ **T/F: Generally speaking, athletes should follow the same dietary lipid guidelines as the general population.**

True. Recommendations for dietary lipid intake for athletes generally follow prudent recommendations for the general population.

❏❏ **Identify four fat soluble vitamins.**

Vitamins A, D, E, K.

❏❏ **Identify four food sources, rich in protein.**

Good sources of protein are eggs, milk, poultry, meat, grains and legumes. However grains and legumes do not provide a full complement of essential amino acids.

❏❏ **Athletes in training have increased protein needs. A study examining the protein requirements of experienced resistance – training athletes found that those consuming the RDA for protein (0.8g/kg/d) had a negative nitrogen balance. How much protein intake would you recommend to an adult athlete in order to maintain a zero balance?**

1.4 g/kg/day.

❏❏ **T/F: Proteins are used in the body to build muscle. They have no role in energy production as an energy substrate.**

False. Although most fuel comes from carbohydrates, both fats and proteins do provide some source of energy. In particular, alanine is synthesized by active skeletal muscle from pyruvate. After four hours of continuous light exercise, the liver's output of alanine derived glucose accounts for about 45% of the liver's total glucose release.

❑❑ **A free radical is a highly reactive molecular fragment that is known to be produced by oxygen consumption. These entities are thought to increase the potential for cellular damage as a result of oxidative stress. This stress may be reduced by the use of antioxidant vitamins. Identify vitamins, which are antioxidants.**

Vitamin C, Vitamin E and beta carotene.

❑❑ **What is a nutraceutical?**

Neutraceuticals are foods or parts of foods that provide medical or health benefits including prevention and/ or treatment of disease.

❑❑ **T/F: Excess fat soluble vitamins accumulate in body tissues and can become toxic.**

True.

❑❑ **What is the most common mineral deficiency in the United States?**

Iron. Although deficiencies of the other minerals may be seen, iron is by far the most common mineral that may be deficient. Selenium deficiency is extremely rare in this country.

❑❑ **T/F: Vitamin supplementation above the RDA has not been demonstrated to improve athletic performance.**

True.

❑❑ **T/F: Vitamins are important in the regulation of metabolism and energy release.**

True.

❑❑ **What is the most important factor in the prevention of bone loss with age?**

Adequate calcium intake. Although regular exercise, avoidance of cigarette smoking, avoiding excess protein intake and excessive alcohol intake are also important in minimizing the risks of bone loss, the most important defense is adequate calcium intake.

❑❑ **Magnesium plays a vital role in many bodily functions, including glucose metabolism, proper neuromuscular function and serving as a cofactor in many chemical reactions. The ingestion of separate magnesium supplements is not recommended. Why?**

Separate magnesium preparations often are mixed with dolomite, which is an extract of limestone and marble. This combination contains the toxic elements mercury and lead.

❏❏ **Athletes have a higher plasma volume. Consequently, when measuring hemoglobin to determine the possibility of iron deficiency the actual number may be factitiously low. What is the most accurate way to determine iron deficiency in an athlete?**

The most accurate method of determining the actual occurrence of iron deficiency in an athlete is by measurement of serum ferritin.

❏❏ **T/F: As a result of excessive sweating in the healthy athlete, minerals are lost at an accelerated rate. This results in a marked increase in the recommended daily requirement of certain minerals, in particular sodium.**

False. Although excessive sweating does increase the loss of water and minerals, it does not increase the mineral requirements above recommended levels in the healthy athlete.

❏❏ **How is obesity defined in terms of Body Mass Index?**

Obesity is defined as Body Mass Index (BMI) ≥ 30 kg/m^2.

❏❏ **How is overweight defined?**

Overweight is defined as a Body Mass Index between 25.0 and 29.9 kg/m^2.

❏❏ **T/F: Unlike medications, dietary supplements are presumed safe until the FDA receives multiple reports of adverse events.**

True.

❏❏ **Nutritional status is an important factor in wound healing. At what level of malnutrition is a significant impact seen on wound healing?**

Severe malnutrition with serum protein levels below 2 gms%.

❏❏ **Which other nutritional deficiencies are also associated with deficient wound healing?**

Vitamin C deficiency.
Severe elemental Zinc deficiency.

❏❏ **What is the heat of combustion?**

The heat of combustion is the heat liberated by oxidizing a specific food; in other words, the food's energy value.

❏❏ **Why does lipid oxidation produce greater energy than protein and carbohydrate oxidation (Fats produce 9 cal/kg, carbohydrates and protein 4 cal/kg)?**

Lipids have more hydrogen atoms available for cleavage and oxidation.

❑❑ What should a pre-competition meal include and why?

A pre-competition should be high in complex carbohydrates, low in fats and protein and high in water content. Further, avoid foods that may spoil if left unrefrigerated for several hours. The meal should be psychologically pleasing to the athlete (familiar foods that contribute to good performance). This may be a special food or appropriate food. It provides energy for filling carbohydrate stores in the liver and muscles, optimizes hydration status; Carbohydrates are digested more rapidly than fats and protein. Protein digestion produces nitrogen; in excess the nitrogen is excreted through the kidney, resulting in relative water depletion through urination. Fats are slow to leave the stomach and give the athlete a " heavy sensation".

❑❑ When should the precompetition meal be eaten?

Ideally three hours before activity to allow for proper digestion and stomach emptying. One can eat closer to competition, but the athlete should select foods that are easily digested.

❑❑ What is the longest interval an athlete should go without eating?

Six hours is a general guideline for anyone to go without ingestion of food.

❑❑ What is the best time for reloading glycogen stores following exhaustive exercise?

The body is most receptive to restoring glycogen stores immediately after activity. The first 30 minutes, the first two hours, the first eight hours are key time periods when the body is most able to replenish glycogen in muscles. Athletes should eat carbohydrate rich foods as soon after activity as possible (allowing for their personal ability to digest foods after activity). More specifically, 1.5 g/kg of carbohydrates within 30 minutes of exercise and an additional 1.5 g/kg within 2 hours of exercise. Since glycogen stores replenish at an average rate of 5% to 7% per hour, it takes at least 20 hours to *fully* re-establish glycogen stores after a glycogen- depleting bout of exercise.

❑❑ For an athlete at an away game, what are some foods that an athlete could carry in their travel bag that could help replenish glycogen stores?

Bananas, oranges, boxes of fruit juices, raisins, bagels, carrots.

❑❑ What are the three main factors responsible for the prevention of osteoporosis?

Calcium intake, circulating estrogen levels and physical activity. In the premenopausal woman, circulating estrogen is the most dominant factor of the three. While adequate calcium intake is crucial and physical activity helpful, in the absence of regular menstrual cycles (adequate estrogen), even the intake of adequate calcium will not maintain normal bone density. In the postmenopausal woman at high risk for osteoporosis, consideration should be given to estrogen replacement therapy in addition to calcium intake and physical activity.

❐❐ **What three roles does estrogen play in maintaining bone health?**

Increases intestinal absorption of calcium, reduced urinary calcium excretion and facilitates calcium retention by bone.

❐❐ **What are the three components of the female athlete triad?**

Disordered eating, amenorrhea and osteoporosis.

❐❐ **Name several features or characteristics associated with the female athlete triad.**

Adolescent or young adult, multiple or recurrent stress fractures, lean and low body mass, compulsive behavior, highly competitive, low self esteem, perfectionist, self critical, depression.

❐❐ **What are several behaviors associated with disordered eating?**

Preoccupation with food, calories and weight; increasing criticism of one's body; secretly eating or stealing food; wide weight fluctuations over a short period of time; severe caloric restrictions; excessive use of laxatives; compulsive, excessive exercise; unwillingness to eat in front of others; wearing baggy, layered clothes; frequent drinking of diet soda or water.

❐❐ **Which diagnostic test is considered the gold standard for assessing bone density?**

DEXA - dual energy x-ray absorptiometry.

❐❐ **How is caloric restriction related to amenorrhea and to bone density?**

The combination of weight loss, low body fat and poor nutrition blunt estrogen synthesis by peripheral fat. Coupled with exercise/ training- induced hormonal alterations as well as physical and psychological stress, a hypothalamic – pituitary dysfunction occurs, leading in turn to amenorrhea. Since bone density is closely related to menstrual regularity and the total number of menstrual cycles, cessation of regular menstrual cycles removes estrogen's protective effect on bone density.

❐❐ **What is considered to be the minimal daily caloric intake recommended for females to dramatically reduce the risk of the female athlete triad?**

2500 calories. Under no circumstances should a female athlete ingest less than 1500 calories, her basal metabolism rate.

❐❐ **Name several food sources rich in calcium.**

Milk (300mg/ 8 0z), milk products – low-fat plain yogurt (415mg) and cheddar cheese (204 mg/1 oz); calcium fortified orange juice (250 mg/ glass); sardines (326 mg/3 oz); canned salmon (167 mg/3 oz); kidney beans (90 mg / cup); almonds (1273 mg/4 oz; and leafy green vegetables (280 mg/ cup).

❏❏ **What is the recommended daily intake of calcium for athletic adolescent girls?**

1500 mg/ day; for middle aged women 1200 – 1500 mg/ day.

❏❏ **What is the Respiratory Quotient (RQ)? What information does it provide?**

The respiratory quotient (RQ) is the ratio of carbon dioxide produced to oxygen consumed. The respiratory quotient provides information about the nutrient mixture catabolized.

❏❏ **What is the respiratory quotient (RQ) for carbohydrates, lipids and proteins?**

The respiratory quotient for carbohydrates is 1.0, for lipids 0.70 and protein 0.82

❏❏ **Name the major categories of the food guide pyramid and the daily recommended number of servings from each category.**

Bread, cereals, rice and pasta: 6 – 11 servings.
Vegetable group: 3 – 5 servings.
Fruit groups: 2-4 servings.
Milk, yogurt, cheese group: 2- 3 servings.
Meat, poultry, fish, dry beans, eggs and nuts group: 2 – 3 servings.
Fats, oils and sweets: use sparingly.

❏❏ **What percentage of caloric intake should come from carbohydrates, protein and lipids?**

Carbohydrates: 55 -60%.
Lipids (fats): < 30%.
Proteins: < 15 – 20%.
The fat recommendation for athletes should be closer to 20 – 25%, increasing carbohydrates towards 60 – 65%.

❏❏ **What is the glycemic index?**

The glycemic index provides a relative (quantitative) indicator of an ingested carbohydrate's ability to raise blood glucose levels. It is determined after ingesting 50 grams of carbohydrate and comparing it over a two hour period to a " standard " for carbohydrate, usually white bread or glucose itself. These two items have an assigned value of 100.

❏❏ **What is the relevance of glycemic index to athletes?**

For athletes who seek to replenish glycogen stores after strenuous activity, or maintain freshness during a day long tournament, and when events are scheduled over several days, knowledge of the glycemic index of foods is important.

❏❏ **What physiologic circulatory parameters affect the glycemic index?**

Glucose transport into cells is facilitated by (1) the hormonal milieu reflected by elevated insulin; (2) the increased tissue sensitivity to insulin and other glucose transporter compounds; (3) low catecholamine levels; (4) increased activity of a specific form of glycogen storing enzyme, glycogen synthetase.

❏❏ Name several common high and moderate glycemic foods.

Carrots (92), honey (87), corn flakes (80), whole meal bread (72), new potatoes (70), raisins (64), bananas (62), corn (59), pasta (50), oatmeal (49), oranges (40).

❏❏ Are high glycemic index foods good choices for pre exercise feedings (within 30 minutes of competition)?

No. The ideal meal immediately before exercising should provide a source of glucose to maintain blood sugar and muscle metabolism with a minimal increase in insulin release. High insulin release just prior to activity will result in a sharp drop in blood sugar just as the athlete begins to work out.

❏❏ What is the heat of combustion?

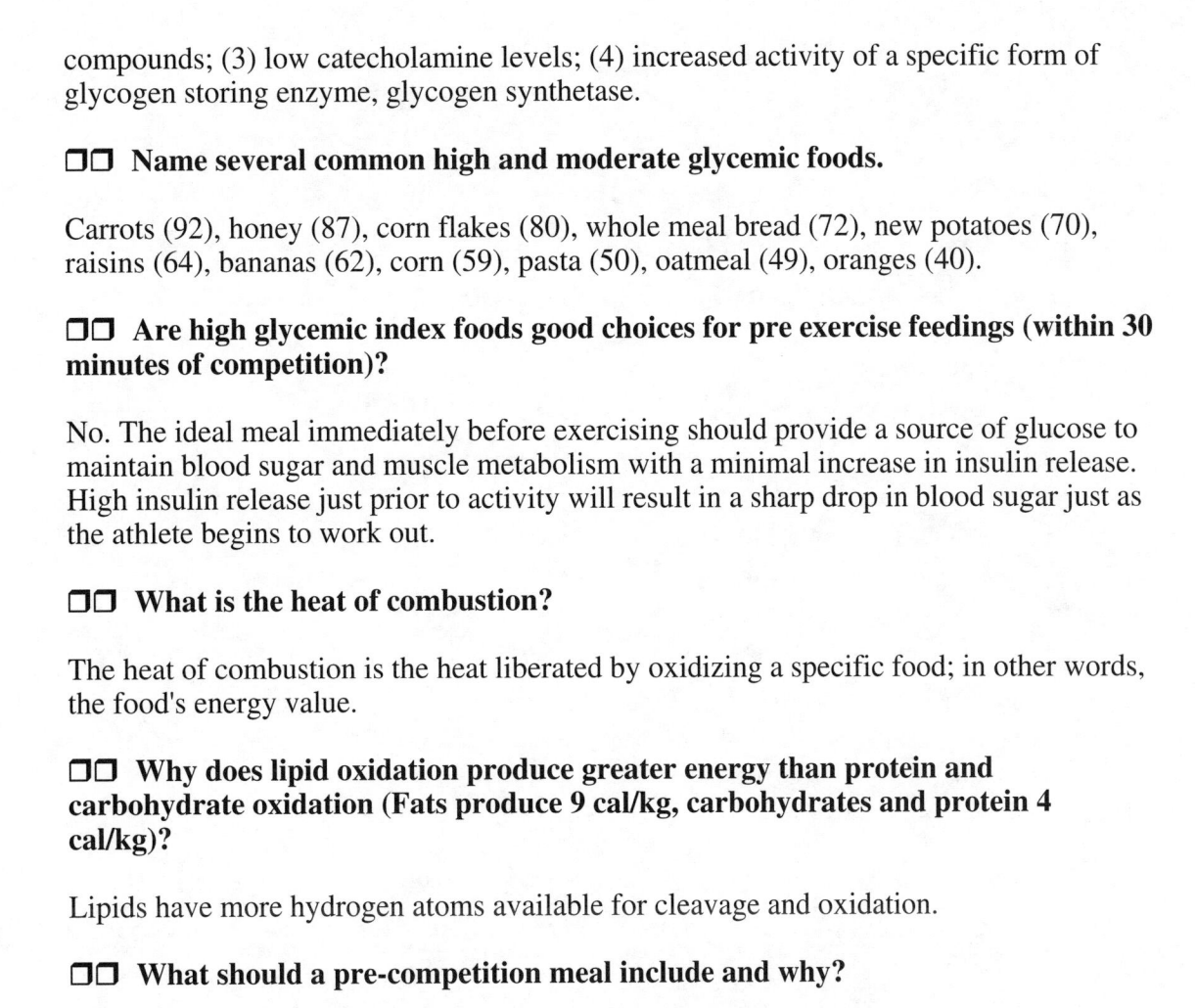

The heat of combustion is the heat liberated by oxidizing a specific food; in other words, the food's energy value.

❏❏ Why does lipid oxidation produce greater energy than protein and carbohydrate oxidation (Fats produce 9 cal/kg, carbohydrates and protein 4 cal/kg)?

Lipids have more hydrogen atoms available for cleavage and oxidation.

❏❏ What should a pre-competition meal include and why?

A pre-competition meal should be high in complex carbohydrates, low in fats and protein, and high in water content. Further, avoid foods that may spoil if left unrefrigerated for several hours. The meal should be psychologically pleasing to the athlete (familiar foods that contribute to good performance). This may be a special food or appropriate food. It provides energy for filling carbohydrate stores in the liver and muscles, optimizes hydration status; Carbohydrates are digested more rapidly than fats and protein. Protein digestion produces nitrogen; in excess the nitrogen is excreted through the kidney, resulting in relative water depletion through urination. Fats are slow to leave the stomach and give the athlete a "heavy sensation".

CLINICAL SPORTS MEDICINE

PREPARTICIPATION PHYSICAL EXAMINATION

❏❏ **Of all athletes screened in a preparticipation physical examination, the number that fails to qualify for participation is:**

Only 0.3-1.9% of athletes screened fail to qualify.

❏❏ **What is the main objective of the Preparticipation Physical examination (PPE)?**

The main objective of the PPE is to detect conditions that would place an athlete at risk for injury, disability or death.

❏❏ **List three secondary objectives of the PPE.**

1. Determining general health.
2. Assessing fitness levels for specific sports.
3. Enabling physicians to counsel on health-related issues are all objectives of the PPE.

❏❏ **T/F: An objective of the PPE is to satisfy legal or insurance requirements.**

True.

❏❏ **What is the optimal timing for the PPE?**

The optimal timing of the PPE is four to six weeks before preseason practice. This allows for scheduling conflicts and to address any injuries or concerns.

❏❏ **T/F: The NCAA requires only one PPE when entering a school's athletic program.**

True.

❏❏ **Name three disadvantages of doing the PPE in a physician office setting.**

It is expensive; it is time consuming for the physician, and it is inconvenient for physician and athlete because of the number of athletes needing to be screened.

❏❏ **List three advantages of the station examination for the PPE.**

A large number of athletes can be screened in a relatively short amount of time; it is cost effective for health care providers and many unique skills of health care providers (physical therapists, athletic trainers, dentists, dietitians, etc) can be used.

❏❏ **Name a disadvantage of the station examination for the PPE.**

The providers do not know the athletes they are screening.

❏❏ **T/F: All of the following tests are recommended as part of the PPE: Urinalysis, complete blood count, and electrocardiogram.**

False. None of the above tests are recommended for routine screening.

❏❏ **T/F: Screening echocardiograms are very effective at identifying conditions that affect clearance.**

False. In a 1995 study, Weidenbener, et al, incorporated echocardiography into the PPE. Of the nearly 3000 exams, no conditions were found effecting clearance.

❏❏ **T/F: Exercise induced asthma is a very commonly undiagnosed ailment.**

True.

❏❏ **List four risk factors for HIV and hepatitis.**

Multiple sex partners, blood transfusions before 1985, history of IV drug abuse and females with male bisexual partners

❏❏ **What percentage of problems can be identified by a good medical history?**

Approximately 75% of all problems affecting athletes can be identified from a good history.

❏❏ **T/F: Many over-the-counter supplements contain substances that are banned by the NCAA or United States Olympic Committee.**

True.

❏❏ **T/F: Over 95% of all sudden deaths in athletes under age 30 are due to structural cardiac abnormalities.**

True.

❏❏ **What number of high school athletes per academic year will suffer from sudden cardiac death?**

1 in 200,000.

❏❏ **Name four risk factors for heat illness.**

Use of antihistamines or stimulants, prior heat illness, poor exercise tolerance and obesity.

❏❏ **List four "groups" of athletes at risk for eating disorders.**

Athletes involved in weight classes (i.e. wrestling or rowing), athletes involved in sports where size is imperative (i.e. football or sumo wrestling), athletes involved in sports where there is emphasis on leanness (i.e. running, swimming), and athletes involved in sports where there in emphasis on appearance (gymnastics, diving, figure skating)

❏❏ **What is the approximate ratio of female to male eating disorders?**

The female to male ratio of eating disorders is approximately 10:1.

❏❏ **T/F: Nicotine has been shown to improve athletic performance.**

False.

❏❏ **T/F: The best way to avoid transmission of HIV and other STD's is sexual abstinence.**

True.

❏❏ **T/F: Anabolic steroids have been shown to be a risk factor for myocardial infarction.**

True.

❏❏ **T/F: The use of the body mass index (BMI) may help to identify overly thin or obese individuals.**

True.

❏❏ **Name four drugs which can cause elevated blood pressure.**

Caffeine, cocaine, nicotine, and ephedrine are all stimulants and can lead to elevated blood pressure.

❏❏ **T/F: A 1/6 systolic heart murmur does not require further evaluation prior to clearance for sports participation**

True. 1/6 systolic murmurs are very common and do not require further evaluation.

❏❏ **T/F: Diastolic heart murmurs require further evaluation prior to clearance for sports participation.**

True.

❏❏ **At what intensity would a heart murmur definitely require further evaluation prior to clearance for sports participation (i.e. 1/6, 2/6, or 3/6).**

3/6.

❏❏ **T/F: The PPE may be an ideal setting and opportunity to educate male athletes on self-testicular examination.**

True.

❏❏ **T/F: Tanner staging is no longer recommended as part of the PPE.**

True.

❏❏ **T/F: It has been reported that not making a team had a greater impact on the lives of young athletes than the death of a friend, separation of parents or a failing grade in school.**

True.

❏❏ **List four conditions associated with mitral valve prolapse that will prevent sports participation.**

History of arrhythmia with syncope, family history of sudden death thought to be related to MVP, history of embolic event and moderate to severe mitral regurgitation.

❏❏ **T/F: Athletes with firmly diagnosed hypertrophic cardiomyopathy (HCM) should not be given clearance for athletic participation, with the possible exception of low-intensity sports.**

True.

❏❏ **T/F: Marked right ventricular hypertrophy is attributed to morbidity and mortality of hypertrophic cardiomyopathy.**

False. Marked left ventricular hypertrophy is associated with HCM morbidity and mortality.

❏❏ **Name three distinct components of hypertrophic cardiomyopathy that are attributed to morbidity and mortality.**

Marked left ventricular hypertrophy, basal outflow obstruction and atrial fibrillation.

☐☐ **T/F: Athletes with best correctable vision 20/40 should wear protective eye wear?**

True.

☐☐ **T/F: Athletes with an inguinal hernia may not participate in any sport.**

False. Symptomatic inguinal hernias should be restricted from participation, but asymptomatic hernias may be corrected after the season or when they become symptomatic.

☐☐ **T/F: Undescended testicles require further evaluation and carry a higher risk for testicular cancer.**

True.

☐☐ **Name the most common respiratory problem (excluding infection) in young athletes that affects participation**

Exercise induced asthma.

☐☐ **Define a concussion.**

Traumatic alteration in mental status.

☐☐ **List four common signs or symptoms of the postconcussion syndrome?**

Headache, mental confusion, dizziness, nausea, irritability, impaired memory and difficulty concentrating.

☐☐ **T/F: Any athlete with a history of transient quadriplegia requires further evaluation with consideration for referral to a neurosurgeon.**

True.

☐☐ **T/F: HIV is more virulent than Hepatitis B.**

False. Hepatitis B is present at concentrations of 100 million per milliliter, compared to a few hundred or thousands with HIV.

☐☐ **T/F: Athletes with sickle cell trait should not participate in sports.**

False. In athletes with sickle cell trait, less than half of hemoglobin is affected and these individuals have no associated anemia. Generally, there are no restrictions. Carriers of the trait, however, should avoid extremes of training (heat/hydration), as they may be at an increased risk for rhabdomyolysis.

❏❏ **List two common most common congenital disabilities of Special Olympic athletes.**

The most common disabilities for athletes in Special Olympics include Down's syndrome and cerebral palsy.

❏❏ **T/F: Down's syndrome carries no athletic restrictions, as these athletes have mental disabilities, not physical.**

False. Athletes with Down's syndrome may also have atlanto-axial instability, cardiac abnormalities, or other congenital abnormalities that may limit athletic participation.

❏❏ **What are the Paralympics?**

The Olympic Games for physically disabled athletes.

❏❏ **Name the three main components of the female athlete triad.**

The female athlete triad includes amenorrhea, eating disorder, and osteoporosis.

❏❏ **Name five negative side effects from using anabolic steroids.**

Anabolic steroid use may cause testicular atrophy, gynecomastia, liver damage, cholesterol elevation, acne, hirsutism, menstrual changes, closure of growth plate, sudden death, and male pattern baldness.

❏❏ **T/F: Wrestling is considered a contact/collision sport.**

True. Wrestling is considered a contact/collision sports.

❏❏ **T/F: Pole vaulting and skiing are considered non-contact sports.**

False. Pole vault and skiing are limited contact sports.

❏❏ **T/F: Cardiovascular abnormalities are the leading causes for restriction from participation?**

False. Musculoskeletal abnormalities, not cardiovascular abnormalities lead to the majority of sports restrictions.

❏❏ **List three signs of Marfan's syndrome.**

Marfan's should be considered with a positive family history, cardiac murmur or click, kyphoscoliosis, pectus excavatum, myopia, ectopic lens, and arm span greater than height.

❏❏ **T/F: Carditis precludes athletic participation.**

True.

❑❑ **T/F: Diabetes mellitus precludes any athletic participation.**

False. If diabetes is under control, athletic participation is allowed.

❑❑ **T/F: Hepatomegaly precludes participation in contact sports.**

True. Hepatomegaly precludes participation in contact/collision sports, but is allowed in non-contact sports.

❑❑ **T/F: The PPE is not complete until a thorough social history is obtained.**

False. The PPE does not require a complete social history, but as time and privacy allow, this should be included. The PPE is an excellent opportunity to cover issues of sexuality, smoking, alcohol use, and substance abuse. Many athletes use the PPE for their health maintenance exam, and these issues are not addressed elsewhere. If unable to address these important issues during the PPE, the athlete should be referred to his/her primary physician for a health maintenance exam.

❑❑ **Name two reasons that recent illness, diarrhea or fever is significant in the setting of the PPE.**

Recent illness, diarrhea, or fever would preclude clearance for participation until the athlete is well. Organomegaly may lead to risk of rupture in contact/collision sports. Fever may lead to dehydration.

❑❑ **T/F: Antibiotic use is important in determining clearance for participation.**

False. Antibiotics play no role in determining clearance.

❑❑ **Why is family history important in the medical history for the PPE?**

Family history is important because certain genetic conditions can be inherited by offspring leading to morbidity or mortality.

❑❑ **What is the ratio of males to females for sudden cardiac death.**

The correct ratio of males to females for sudden cardiac death is 5 to 1.

❑❑ **T/F: Athletes should never be disqualified for a dermatologic condition.**

False. Temporary restriction may be imposed on athletes with tinea, herpes simplex, scabies, lice, molluscum contagiosum, impetigo, or warts until treatment is completed. This applies mainly to contact sports or where use of mats or equipment may contribute to transmission. Athletes may be permitted to participate if a lesion is adequately covered.

❑❑ **T/F: Burners and stingers often result in permanent disability?**

False. Burners and stingers rarely result in permanent deficits. Associated numbness, pain, or weakness generally resolves in minutes.

❑❑ **Approximately 5,000 young people take their lives in the U.S. yearly. How many attempts at suicide are made for every death?**

The correct answer is 50 to 200.

❑❑ **What percentage of AIDS cases occur between the ages of 20 to 25?**

21% of AIDS cases occur between the ages of 20 to 25, with acquisition during adolescents (based on incubation period).

❑❑ **Name three components of the cardiovascular portion of the PPE.**

Precordial auscultation on standing and supine position, palpation of femoral artery pulses and brachial blood pressure in the sitting position. Femoral artery asymmetry may indicate coarctation. Standing and sitting auscultation can help to identify dynamic left ventricular outflow obstruction.

❑❑ **Describe the Valsalva maneuver to help characterizing cardiac murmurs.**

Valsalva reduces venous return, increasing obstruction and the intensity of the murmur in hypertrophic cardiomyopathy. With aortic stenosis, Valsalva reduces the murmur (by reducing venous return), while squatting increases the murmur (by increasing venous return). Innocent murmurs act similarly to aortic stenosis.

❑❑ **Name three purposes of the general screening musculoskeletal examination portion of the PPE.**

The general screening examination is a tool used to quickly determine range of motion, gross motor function, and significant injury.

❑❑ **List three injuries that female athletes who participate in soccer and basketball are particularly susceptible to.**

Patellofemoral syndrome, stress fractures and anterior cruciate ligament injuries.

❑❑ **List the three categories of clearance determination.**

Unrestricted, dependent on further evaluation or rehabilitation, and no clearance for a given sport or any sport.

❑❑ **T/F: Athletes with mild to moderate hypertension, without end-organ damage, may participate in all levels of competition.**

True.

❑❑ **T/F: Athletes taking anti-hypertensive medications should not participate in athletics.**

False.

CLINICAL SPORTS MEDICINE

CONDITIONING AND TRAINING

☐☐ **T/F: Deconditioning and detraining occur at similar rates in the adult and the preadolescent athlete.**

True.

☐☐ **T/F: Resistance training in skeletally immature athletes has an adverse impact on linear growth.**

False.

☐☐ **T/F: Physical training and conditioning programs that includes vigorous aerobic components may increase linear growth in skeletally immature athletes.**

True. Vigorous conditioning programs promotes endogenous growth hormone production and release and consequently enhances linear growth potential in skeletally immature athletes.

☐☐ **T/F: Strength training is a useful component in management of obesity in young females.**

False. Strength training has, at a minimum, no positive effect on total body fat reduction and may actually increase certain subsets of adipose tissue in certain populations.

☐☐ **T/F: The degree of improvement in body composition and muscular strength following resistance training is independent of an athlete's body build.**

False. Body build significantly affects the degree of alteration in body composition following resistance training.

☐☐ **T/F: Hypertension is a contraindication to initiating strength and conditioning programs.**

False. Patients with severe, uncontrolled hypertension should refrain from including Olympic lifts and maximal lifts in their training regimen. Likewise, if a patient is at risk for hypotensive syncopal complications of medications used to treat hypertension, modification of training regimen may be required.

☐☐ **Can resistance training improve hemodynamics in hypertensive adolescents?**

Weight training, when combined with a balanced training regimen that includes endurance training, improves blood pressure in hypertensive adolescents.

❑❑ **T/F: Hypertension is an expected finding in adults for one to two hours after moderate to heavy exercise.**

False. Hypotension is the expected physiological response after exercise.

❑❑ **T/F: Children with asthma can improve their work and exercise tolerance with an exercise program that includes endurance training.**

True.

❑❑ **In both children and adults, which parameter is more predictive of athletic performance, VO$_2$Max or Anaerobic threshold?**

Anaerobic threshold.

❑❑ **Which metabolic pathway is utilized by muscle cells for intense periods of exercise lasting one to two minutes in duration?**

Anaerobic glycolysis.

❑❑ **In calculating a MET in an exercising athlete, one MET is 3.6ml/kg/min. What is the ml a measure of?**

Ml of Oxygen consumed.

❑❑ **T/F: A decreased resting heart rate is a sign of overtraining in endurance athletes.**

False. Resting heart rate is an unreliable marker in overtraining in both endurance and non-endurance sports.

❑❑ **In the glycolysis biochemical pathway, which enzyme is the predominant rate limiting enzyme.**

Phosphofructokinase.

❑❑ **Interval training or interval sprinting is utilized in training regimens to increase which parameter, endurance or power?**

Endurance.

❑❑ **Which sub-type of muscle fibers predominate in "power" athletes, utilize anaerobic metabolic pathways, and are innervated by high threshold neurons?**

Type Iib.

❑❑ **Which type of muscle fibers are "fast twitch" and are important in athletes who require both speed and endurance components for competition?**

Type Iia.

❐❐ **T/F: Type I muscle fibers are the muscle fibers utilized in endurance sports.**

True. These "slow twitch" fibers have higher levels of myoglobin and more resistance to fatigue in endurance events.

❐❐ **T/F: The ratio of muscle fiber types and subtypes cannot be altered by training, the profile of muscle fiber types in an individual athlete is determined exclusively by genetics.**

False. Training and detraining can especially affect the transition of muscle fiber subtypes from one type to the next.

❐❐ **T/F: GABA (gamma aminobutyric acid) is a neurotransmitter that is inhibitory to muscled contraction.**

True.

❐❐ **T/F: The amount of time that it takes for an athlete to acclimatize to a specific altitude depends only on the physiological characteristics of the athlete.**

False. The amount of time required to acclimatize also depends on the specific altitude. Higher altitudes require longer periods of acclimatization.

❐❐ **T/F: Individual human muscle cells generate equivalent amounts of force in males and females.**

True.

❐❐ **T/F: VO_2 max decreases with age.**

True. Decreases range from 0.3 to 0.5 ml/min/kg/year.

❐❐ **Which two parameters that influence VO_2 are increased by training.**

Maximum cardiac output and maximal arteriovenous oxygen difference.

❐❐ **What are three EKG findings that constitute a "positive" exercise stress test?**

1. Horizontal or downsloping ST depression greater than or equal to 1mm @ 80 ms.
2. Upsloping ST depression greater than or equal to 1.5 mm @ 80 ms.
3. Horizontal or upsloping ST elevation greater than or equal to 1.5mm @ 80 ms.

❐❐ **T/F: Thrombophlebitis is a contraindication to graded exercise testing.**

True.

❐❐ **T/F: Endurance is improved in strength training regimens with resistance at loads of 60-70% of one RepMax.**

True.

❑❑ **T/F: A single exercise session can have a positive effect on improving clinical depression.**

True.

❑❑ **T/F: The positive effects of exercise on depression are limited to the duration of the exercise session.**

False. The amelioration of clinical depression symptoms persists beyond the end of the exercise session.

❑❑ **T/F: Exercise has a greater effect on depression in female patients when compared with the effect of exercise in depressed male patients.**

False. The positive effect of exercise on depression is equal in male and female subjects.

❑❑ **Rate the following modalities as to their effectiveness in decreasing depression: exercise alone, exercise combined with psychotherapy, psychotherapy alone.**

An Exercise program, when combined with psychotherapy, is the most effective modality of the three listed. Exercise alone is more effective than psychotherapy alone.

❑❑ **T/F: The amount of muscle required to lift a weight is less in the trained muscle than in the untrained muscle.**

True. This physiologic fact is a factor in the need for an athlete to progressively increase the amount of resistance in order to continue to gain strength.

❑❑ **T/F: Adaptations in progressive resistance training show greater changes in the neuro-muscular junction late (after 8 weeks of exercise) in the exercise phase.**

False. Changes at the neuromuscular junctions are most obvious in the early phases (2-8 weeks) of an exercise program. Similarly, increased voluntary activation of muscle is the largest contributor to strength increasing in the early phases of resistance training.

❑❑ **At what time interval in a strength training program do muscle hypertrophy factors exceed neuromuscular adaptations as the most significant factor in strength gains?**

After ten weeks of consistent resistance training.

❑❑ **What effect does resistance training have on Type IIb muscle fibers?**

Type IIb muscle fibers constitute a pool of muscle fibers that, with increased resistance training, improve in oxidative ability and begin transformation in their histochemical characteristics that approximate the characteristics of Type IIa fibers.

❑❑ **Changes in muscle fiber morphology have a positive effect on performance after what period of training?**

Three months.

☐☐ **What changes in the muscle result in muscle hypertrophy?**

Increase in the size and number of myofibrils, remodeling of protein within the muscle cell, increase in the number of actin filaments and to a lesser degree myosin filaments all contribute to muscle hypertrophy.

☐☐ **T/F: The number of capillaries supplying blood to a given unit of muscle has been documented to increase with heavy resistance training?**

True.

☐☐ **T/F: The gains in strength and decreases in perceived fatigue that an athlete experiences in exercise are both improved by increased capillary blood flow. This improvement is due exclusively to increased oxygen availability to the muscle unit.**

False. The increased capillary blood flow not only improves the oxygen available to the muscle unit, it also improves lactic acid clearance.

☐☐ **Which factors affect peak force and power output in a contracting muscle?**

Muscle fiber size and length, angle and physical properties of the fiber-tendon attachment to bone, muscle fiber type, and variables in the actin-myosin crossbridge.

☐☐ **T/F: Isometric and isotonic muscle contractile properties are independent of muscle temperature.**
False. Contractile properties are highly dependent on muscle temperature.

☐☐ **T/F: Endurance training results in significant increases in muscle hypertrophy, especially in Type II fibers.**

False. These changes are associated with resistance training.

CLINICAL SPORTS MEDICINE

EXERCISE BENEFITS AND WRITING AN EXERCISE PRESCRIPTION

❑❑ **What is the most common reason for not exercising?**

Lack of time.

❑❑ **What is the physician's responsibility regarding exercise advice?**

The physician should encourage regular exercise as a life style change because almost half of all deaths in the United States may be due to lack of physical activity.

❑❑ **Should all adults over age 30 consult with a physician before starting an exercise program?**

No. Patients do not need to see a physician if they plan a moderate exercise program. However, if the patient plans a vigorous program (> 60% of personal maximum oxygen consumption) or, if the patient has a chronic illness, they should see their physician for medical clearance.

❑❑ **What is the minimum amount of exercise an adult should have?**

Thirty minutes of moderate intensity (i.e. 3-6 mets; up to 50% VO2 max) physical activity on most days of the week. Intermittent bouts of activity (i.e. 10 minutes at a time) accumulated throughout the day is acceptable according to the 1995 CDC/ACSM guidelines. Flexibility and muscle strengthening exercises are additional components that should be encouraged. Despite a nearly 60% success rate in reaching the goals of the Healthy People 2000 initiative which began in 1990, the objectives for increasing physical activity were not met. Indeed the Healthy People 2000 " report card " revealed a decrease in physical activity levels in the past decade and a rise in the number of overweight Americans.

❑❑ **What are the benefits of regular exercise?**

Lowered risk of all cause and cardiovascular mortality; reduction of body fat; improved psychological state; and resistance to stress, injury and disease (coronary artery disease; type II diabetes mellitus; osteoporosis; hypertension; colorectal; prostate and breast cancer). HDL cholesterol rises, triglycerides fall and glucose tolerance is improved with regular physical exercise.

❏❏ **T/F: Only vigorous physical activity confers health benefits.**

False. Moderate exercise will provide health benefits but will not increase VO_2 max except for those at very low levels of fitness. While exercise health benefits are proportionate to the total amount of minutes exercised or total calories expended, vigorous exercise can trigger musculoskeletal complications and cardiovascular events in some individuals.

❏❏ **What improvements in cardiovascular function are seen with regular physical activity?**

Increased maximal oxygen uptake from both central and peripheral adaptations; lowered minute ventilation; lowered myocardial oxygen demand during exercise; lowered heart rate and blood pressure; increased capillary density in skeletal muscles; increased exercise threshold for the accumulation of lactate; and increased exercise threshold for the onset of symptoms of angina pectoris and claudication.

❏❏ **What is the risk of death during an exercise stress test?**

Less than 0.01% (up to 1 death in 10,000 tests) in various studies. There is no difference in risk of physician and non physician (nurse, physical therapist, exercise physiologist and physician assistant) supervised tests. The risk of death during exercise in the community is < 1 in 700,000.

❏❏ **What are the major signs or symptoms of cardiovascular and pulmonary disease that should be evaluated before rendering an exercise prescription to a patient?**

Pain or discomfort in the chest, neck, jaw or arms especially if related to physical activity; dyspnea at rest or with mild exertion; dyspnea or fatigue with ADLs; dizziness; syncope; ankle edema; orthopnea; PND; palpitations; tachycardia; claudication and heart murmur.

Any of these symptoms alone or in combination should be evaluated before writing an exercise prescription. A finding of one of these must be interpreted in the context of the individual patient since these symptoms/signs are not specific for cardiopulmonary disease.

❏❏ **What factors could contribute to a false negative exercise stress testing when it is used as a preliminary screening before an exercise prescription?**

Normal ECG stress testing has been noted in patients who subsequently experience cardiac complications during exercise. Contributing factors may include inadequate cardiac stress, insufficient ECG lead monitoring, drug therapy that masks anginal pain (eg nitrates), and /or ischemic ST segment changes (eg phenothiazine) and baseline ECG abnormalities (ST depression at rest, LVH, LBBB) that make the exercise ECG uninterpretable.

❏❏ **How do you estimate intensity of training for patients?**

There are several formulas that can be used:
1. Maximum heart rate = 220 - age
   - Low intensity = < 60% max HR
   - Moderate intensity = 60 - 75% max HR
   - High intensity = 75 - 90% max HR
2. Maximum heart rate reserve = maximum HR - resting HR then add desired percentage to the resting HR (Karvonen Formula).
3. Maximum VO2 reserve is calculated in similar fashion as max HR reserve substituting VO_2 for HR. While this is the benchmark for estimating intensity of exercise, it is not feasible in clinical settings.

❏❏ **Using Karvonen's formula, prepare an exercise prescription for a 60-year-old man with a resting HR of 80 bpm who desires a moderate exercise prescription.**

Maximum HR (160) - resting HR (80) = 80
50% of 80 = 40
80 + 40 = 120
Therefore a target HR of 120 would achieve desired moderate intensity program.

❏❏ **What level of resistance training should most patients strive for?**

Two to three days a week; 8 - 10 exercises that condition the major muscle groups; at least one set of 8 - 12 repetitions of each exercise however multiple set regimens may provide greater benefits.

❏❏ **What is the value of the Borg Rating of Perceived Exertion (RPE) scale in regards to exercise prescription?**

RPE may be a useful adjunct for aerobic exercise prescription in that most people prefer to exercise at a moderate VO_2 max (60 - 65%) and RPE at these intensities is consistent (12 - 14 RPE on the 6 - 20 scale).

❏❏ **What is the correlation between maximal oxygen uptake (VO_2 max), maximum heart rate and the RPE scale in regards to the exercise prescription?**

VO_2 max is the accepted criterion measurement of cardiorespiratory fitness, however the costs of obtaining this measurement in terms of equipment and personnel are high. Therefore it is not feasible for most exercise prescriptions. VO_2 max can be estimated with reasonable accuracy during exercise test protocols; the standard error is 7% for these estimates. Relative heart rate measurements (such as heart rate reserve) can underestimate the VO_2 max by 5 - 15%. RPE may be a useful adjunct for aerobic exercise prescription in that most people prefer to exercise at a moderate VO_2 max (60-65%) and RPE at these intensities is consistent (12 - 14 RPE on the 6-20 scale).

❏❏ **What increases when the frequency of exercise is increased above five days per week?**

The risk of injury. The additional gain in VO_2 max is minimal at training levels that exceed 5 days/week while the incidence of injury increases disproportionately.

❑❑ **Which patient groups are particularly at risk for debilitating leg injuries with high impact physical activities (e.g. running and jumping)?**

Overweight elderly patients and unfit women. When starting an exercise program, young women have a two fold higher rate of injury compared to young men; older women four fold higher than older men. Weight training before starting high impact sports might reduce the risk, but this needs to be confirmed in research studies.

❑❑ **What advice about exercise prescription would you give a person of average fitness who is interested in weight reduction?**

Exercise alone without calorie restriction has only a modest effect on fat loss. Calorie restriction will more easily induce an energy deficit than exercise. Studies on weight loss are most successful when dieting and exercise are combined. An exercise program of three days / week, expending at least 250 - 300 kcal per exercise session is suggested as the threshold level for fat loss (30 - 45 min of exercise for an average fit person).

❑❑ **How can improvements in both muscular strength and endurance be balanced?**

Muscle strength is best developed by using heavier weight with few repetitions; muscle endurance is developed by using lighter weight with greater number of repetitions (through increase mitochondria in the active muscles). To improve both, most experts recommend 8-12 repetitions per set, however a lower repetition range (e.g. 6-8) may better optimize strength and power. In older or frailer patients, 10 - 15 repetitions at more moderate weight is recommended to avoid orthopedic injury.

❑❑ **What is the overload principle of training?**

The overload principle states that for the musculoskeletal or cardiopulmonary systems to improve their functions they must be exposed to a load that it is not usually accustomed to handling. Repeated exposure triggers adaptations in those tissues that lead to improved function and capacity.

❑❑ **What are the three components of an exercise prescription?**

An exercise prescription should delineate the intensity, duration and frequency of training. The main objective of exercise prescription is to help an individual achieve change in his/her lifestyle to include regular physical activity.

❑❑ **What should the warm up phase of exercise include?**

The exercise session should begin with a warm up consisting of 5 - 10 minutes of calisthenics type and stretching exercises and 5 - 10 minutes of lead in aerobic exercise (i.e. if running is planned, then 5 - 10 minutes of light jogging, etc.).

❑❑ **What are the benefits of warming up?**

The warm-up may prevent musculoskeletal injury by increasing connective tissue extensibility, improving joint range of motion and enhancing muscular performance.

❑❑ **Why must diabetic patients on insulin be under adequate control before starting an exercise program?**

There are several factors that influence response to exercise. Glucose transport into muscles may be impaired; thus glucose availability as energy for exercise may be inadequate in the poorly controlled diabetic. In response, there may be increased use of free fatty acids resulting in ketone body formation and hyperglycemia. A blood glucose level of > 300mg/dl is a relative contraindication to exercise.

❑❑ **What is the most common problem experienced by diabetic patients who exercise?**

Exercise induced hypoglycemia. This is more common among diabetics on insulin than for those on oral hypoglycemic drugs. Exercise has an insulin like effect (increased insulin sensitivity for regular exercisers) in diabetics who are well controlled. Also insulin absorption from the injection site may be increased with exercise (although this is highly variable from one patient to another).

❑❑ **How can exercise induced hypoglycemia be prevented in diabetic patients?**

For diabetics on insulin, check blood glucose before and after exercise; if below 100 mg/dl ingest 20 - 30 gms of carbohydrate. Avoid exercise during peaks of insulin activity. Consider decreasing insulin doses before exercise if the patient has experienced hypoglycemia with exercise previously. Exercise with supervision if hypoglycemia has been experienced previously. If exercise leads to more optimal diabetes control, consider long term insulin reduction (5 - 10% total daily dose at a time, with further adjustments as needed).

❑❑ **What adverse role does diabetic neuropathy play in exercise?**

Autonomic neuropathy may cause orthostatic hypotension, which can increase the risk of dizziness or syncope, during active exercise or the cool down phase. It can also increase the risk of heat related illness when exercising in hot weather. Heart rate response to exercise may be blunted and coronary ischemia may be silent in those diabetics with autonomic neuropathy. These patients must wear proper footwear for physical activity and practice good foot hygiene (e.g. drying their toes to avoid tinea pedia; applying moisturizer to their feet).

❑❑ **What are the contraindications to strenuous exercise in the diabetic patient?**

Poor control, proliferative retinopathy, neuropathy, nephropathy, cardiovascular disease, microangiopathy.

❑❑ **Which diabetic patients should undergo treadmill testing before starting a moderate intensity exercise program?**

Age > 35 years; type II DM of > 10 years duration; type I DM of > 15 years duration; presence of any additional risk factor for coronary artery disease; presence of retinopathy, nephropathy (including microalbuminuria), peripheral vascular disease or autonomic neuropathy.

❏❏ What benefits of exercise have been documented in patients with pulmonary disease?

The bulk of evidence is from studies of COPD patients, which have documented increased exercise capacity, increased functional states, decreased severity of dyspnea and improved quality of life. These changes may decrease hospitalization but do not prolong life in COPD patients.

❏❏ What are the benefits of pursed lip breathing for pulmonary patients?

Pulmonary patients (COPD, asthma, cystic fibrosis) should be taught pursed lip breathing because it decreases the frequency of respiration, increases tidal volume and improves sense of control for oxygenation and improves sense of control over breathing distress.

❏❏ What criteria should be used for supplemental oxygen during exercise in pulmonary patients?

Supplemental O_2 is indicated for patients with a PaO_2 less than or equal to 55 mm Hg or an SaO_2 of less than or equal to 88% while breathing Room Air. The oxygen flow rate should be adjusted during exercise to keep the SaO_2 greater than or equal to 90% throughout exercise.

❏❏ What is the clinical presentation of exercise induced asthma?

Primarily dyspnea on exertion out of proportion to the physical activity and postexercise cough. Also wheezing, chest tightness and/ or sputum production may be noted by the patient.

❏❏ What are the variables of exercise that contribute to bronchospasm?

Intensity of exercise, i.e. more likely with activities at greater than or equal to 65 - 75% VO_2 max; type of activity, i.e. outdoor running is most likely to trigger > treadmill running > cycling> swimming > walking is the least likely to trigger; continuous activity is more likely to trigger than intermittent exercise; environments of cold, dry air is more likely to trigger than warm, moist air.

❏❏ Is resistance training (weight lifting) contraindicated in hypertensive patients?

No. Resistance training should not be the primary form of exercise for hypertensive patients but is a safe component of a fitness program that first emphasizes endurance exercise. Circuit weight training focused on light weight/ higher number of repetitions (20 - 30 per set) may reduce blood pressure. Avoid Valsalva maneuvers during weight lifting.

❏❏ How much will blood pressure decline in response to an endurance exercise program?

Patients with stage 1 or 2 hypertension (BP = 140 - 179/ 90-109 mm HG) will, on average have a 10 mm reduction in both systolic and diastolic blood pressure. Patients with stage 3 or above hypertension should not begin an exercise program until they achieve blood pressure control through pharmacologic therapy.

❐❐ If a patient has a hypertensive response on an exercise treadmill test should he/she be started on medication to lower blood pressure?

There are no clear guidelines in this situation. A hypertensive response to exercise (systolic rise greater than or equal to 200 mm Hg; any rise in diastolic blood pressure, i.e. diastolic blood pressure should drop or stay the same with exercise) even in the face of normal resting blood pressure has been associated with subsequent development of hypertension. Despite this, stress testing for hypertension screening remains an investigational tool and treatment decisions must be individualized to each patient. Consider at least, lifestyle modification advice for such patients.

❐❐ What assessment must be done before prescribing exercise for patients with peripheral vascular disease (PVD) ?

Assess the distance walked before the onset of claudication and the intensity of the claudication. Assess the patient for coronary artery disease because > 50% of the patients who undergo lower extremity revascularization procedures have concomitant severe coronary artery disease (CAD). Improvements in exercise tolerance (reduced claudication) through gradual exercise training may unmask symptoms of angina pectoris. Attempt to modify all CAD risk factors and prescribe aspirin as primary prevention (if not contraindicated by active peptic ulcer, aspirin sensitivity, active bleeding diathesis or underlying hematologic disorder).

❐❐ What type of exercise should be recommended for a PVD patient?

Walking is the preferred mode of exercise; however non weight bearing activities should be encouraged (arm ergometry, rowing) if walking is impaired by unbearable claudication.

❐❐ Is exercise safe during pregnancy?

Yes. Research studies have not demonstrated differences between sedentary and exercising women in terms of rate of miscarriage, uterine rupture, preterm labor, fetal distress, congenital abnormalities or ability to carry to term. Strenuous exercise may lead to a lighter birth weight but the babies are generally healthy.

❐❐ What are the contraindications to exercise during pregnancy?

Hypertension; preterm rupture of membranes; preterm labor during any prior or the current pregnancy; incompetent cervix/ cerclage; persistent second trimester bleeding; intrauterine growth retardation.

❐❐ Which physical activities are safest during pregnancy?

Only scuba diving is absolutely contraindicated. Encourage swimming and cycling. Weight bearing exercises can be continued during pregnancy but not initiated as a new exercise program during pregnancy. Avoid activities that require balance or have any risk of abdominal trauma (contact sports). Avoid supine exercises after the first trimester (reduces cardiac output).

❏❏ **What recommendations can be made for strength training in children and adolescents?**

Strength training is safe before puberty if the prescription emphasizes sport specific exercises and sets of high repetition at low resistance. Weight lifting for competition, power lifting and bodybuilding should be prohibited. These activities pose an enhanced risk because they involve lifting maximal weight or ballistic movements on the immature skeleton. All strength training programs for children must be supervised.

❏❏ **In prepubescent children, why will strength increase with strength training even though muscle hypertrophy doesn't occur?**

Strength training will increase muscle strength before adolescence independent of changes in muscle size. Neurologic adaptations will improve strength, including (1) increased neural drive (% motor unit activation will increase); (2) increased intrinsic muscle contraction and (3) improved motor skill coordination.

❏❏ **For children with cystic fibrosis, what are the potential benefits of exercise?**

Improved mucus clearance; training of respiratory muscles; improved self-image. Encourage jogging, walking and swimming.

❏❏ **Is age predicted peak heart rate accurate in persons over 65 years of age?**

A measured peak heart rate is preferable to an age predicted peak heart rate when prescribing aerobic exercises for people 65 years of age or older because of variability in peak heart rate observed in this age group. An additional influence on peak heart rate may be medications such as digoxin, beta-blockers and calcium channel blockers, which are more commonly used by elderly patients.

❏❏ **How can elderly patients safely increase their exercise program?**

Initially increase exercise duration rather than intensity. If vigorous exercise is planned an elderly patient should consult a physician first.

❏❏ **What are the benefits of resistance training for the elderly?**

Preserves/enhances muscle strength and endurance. This in turn, decreases likelihood of falls, improves mobility, counteracts muscle weakness and frailty and allows performance of activities of daily living with less effort.

❏❏ **What changes associated with aging may have an impact on an elderly athlete?**

Muscle size and mass decrease 3 - 5% per decade after age 30. Cartilage, tendons and ligaments show increased stiffness that could lead to possible injury. Work of breathing increases 20%. Maximal heart rate decreases by 1 beat per year. Cardiac output decreases 8% per decade. Sedentary elderly patients lose VO_2 max at a rate of 10% per decade.

❏❏ **What should be the focus of the exercise prescription in an osteoporotic patient?**

These patients are at increased risk for stress fracture; therefore, exercise should focus on low impact and low intensity at the outset to minimize the risk. Weight bearing exercise over time, will increase bone mineral density and mass. Resistance training (low weight, high number of repetitions) should be encouraged. Aquatic exercises do not improve bone mineral density.

❏❏ **What are the benefits of supervised exercise for patients who recently suffered a major cardiac event (CABG, PTCA, MI, CHF, etc)?**

Reduces the psychological and physiological deterioration induced by bedrest during the hospitalization. Additional safety of supervising these patients as they return to normal activities of daily living in the community. Helps gauge longer-term prognosis by identifying the subset of cardiac patients with adverse cardiovascular and cognitive signs. Eases the patient and family into ongoing recovery at home after hospital discharge.

❏❏ **What are the stages of cardiac rehabilitation programs?**

Phase I - inpatient.
Phase II - up to 12 weeks of supervised exercise and education (on risk factor modification) after hospital discharge.
Phase III - intermittent ECG/ supervision.
Phase IV - no ECG monitoring/ limited supervision.

❏❏ **During the inpatient recovery after an MI, what should be the target intensity of activities be?**

Heart rate < 120 beats per minute; or heart rate at rest + 20 beats per minute; or rating of perceived exertion < 13 (on the Borg 6 - 20 scale).

❏❏ **How can a safe intensity of exercise for outpatient cardiac patients be established?**

The exercise prescription should identify an exercise intensity that will induce a training effect but not exceed a metabolic load that precipitates angina or ischemia. Most cardiac patients are deconditioned; therefore exercise intensity in the range of 40 - 50% VO_2 reserve will suffice for training effect. Target heart rate is widely used as an index of exercise intensity because VO_2 measurements are not feasible in most clinical settings. Maximum heart rate reserve reasonably estimates VO_2 reserve because heart rate and oxygen consumption are linearly related during aerobic exercise that uses large muscle groups (5 - 15% error). Ischemic ST segment depression, anginal symptoms, arrhythmias, blood pressure rise (target < 240 mmHg systolic; < 110 mm Hg diastolic), and RPE (from 11 - 13) should be factored in on an individual basis (i.e. target heart rate is _not_ the final word for all patients!). Target heart rate should be set at least 10 beats per minute below the heart rate associated with angina or ischemic signs. Patients who experience angina during exercise at aerobic levels < 3 mets are not candidates for an exercise program.

Can information from pharmacological stress testing be applied to the exercise prescription?

Often it cannot. Dipyridamole or adenosine studies with myocardial perfusion imaging and dobutamine echocardiography are being increasingly used but do not provide information on exercise capacity, hemodynamic responses or an ischemic ECG threshold. Dobutamine often induces sinus tachycardia; therefore if no ischemia is noted on the cardiogram, the maximal heart rate during the study can guide target heart rate for the exercise prescription. Otherwise, cardiac patients who have not had a preliminary exercise test must receive a conservative exercise prescription (THR = resting HR + 20 beats / min; 2-3 mets) and be closely monitored.

Should cardiac patients lift weights?

Resistance training will lower the rate pressure product when lifting, thus reducing the cardiac demands during daily activities. Endurance will increase through weight training. Finally, resistance training will increase muscle mass and in turn, basal metabolic rate increases. This may aid the cardiac patient in losing weight for secondary risk factor modification. Low to moderate risk cardiac patients should be encouraged to include weight lifting after a sustained period of supervised aerobic training (at least 2 weeks). However resistance training in female and elderly coronary patients, and those with concomitant severe left ventricular dysfunction has not been adequately studied. In these specific groups caution is advised and weight lifting programs must be gradual and carefully supervised. Cardiac patients should be advised to avoid Valsalva and excessive handgrip when lifting weight (to avoid excessive systolic blood pressure rise). Teach "blow the weights up", e.g. exhale upon lifting and inhale upon lowering.

What physiologic changes effect exercise tolerance in congestive heart failure?

Central hemodynamic changes include reduced cardiac output at rest and /or during exercise, elevated left ventricular filling pressure, ventricular volume overload and elevated central venous and pulmonary pressures. These changes contribute to hyperventilation with exercise, early fatigue and lactate accumulation in the blood even at low intensity exercise. Peripherally, skeletal muscles show maladaptive glycolytic mechanisms that further reduces VO_2 max in CHF patients. While exercise will not improve cardiac output in these patients, it will lead to skeletal muscle adaptations that increase endurance and reduce CHF symptoms.

Which patients are at high risk for cardiac complications during exercise?

Those with unstable angina, severe aortic stenosis, uncontrolled cardiac arrhythmias, decompensated CHF, acute myocarditis or infective endocarditis. These patients should not exercise until the above problems are controlled.

CLINICAL SPORTS MEDICINE

EPIDEMIOLOGY OF SPORTS INJURIES

❑❑ **In the United States which sports are associated with the highest incidence of head injury?**

Football, horseback riding and bicycling, especially in children.

❑❑ **What is the most common brain injury during sports?**

Concussion.

❑❑ **T/F: Most sports related head injuries (except for boxing or combat sports) are accidental.**

True.

❑❑ **T/F: Football players who sustain a concussion are four times more likely to have a subsequent concussion.**

True.

❑❑ **What is the concern about repetitive overhead throwing in skeletally immature pitchers?**

Growth plate stress fractures.

❑❑ **Which sports are associated with medial epicondylitis?**

Baseball, golf and racquetball are examples. This is an overuse syndrome.

❑❑ **T/F: Women runners are more likely to have stress fractures than men.**

Women runners are at increased risk for the development of stress fractures.

❑❑ **List factors felt to play a role in the increased risk for stress fractures in women.**

Age, poor fitness, non-black race, menstrual irregularities.

❑❑ **Name two conditions that predispose the athlete to stress fractures?**

Hyperpronation and tibia vara.

❑❑ **What is the most common foot and ankle injury?**

Ankle sprain.

❑❑ **How do you differentiate a sprain from a strain?**

A sprain is defined as a stretching or tearing of the ligaments, while a strain is defined as an injury to a muscle or tendon.

❑❑ **What is the most common mechanism of injury in clavicle fractures?**

A fall or blow to the point of the shoulder. They are seen most frequently in association with high energy contact sports such as football or hockey or following a fall as in cycling or skiing.

❑❑ **T/F: Distal clavicle osteolysis is most commonly associated with power weight lifters.**

True.

❑❑ **Which sports have been associated with an increase incidence of spondylolysis?**

Gymnastics, diving, wrestling, weightlifting and football.

❑❑ **What is the most common cause of back pain in children and adolescents?**

Spondylolysis.

❑❑ **T/F: Most serious bicycle injuries are the result of collisions with motor vehicles.**

True.

❑❑ **T/F: Wearing bicycle helmets reduces the risk of head injuries by 74 - 85%.**

True.

❑❑ **What is the most common ligament injured in an inversion sprain?**

Anterior talofibular.

❑❑ **What is the most common nerve root affected in sport related brachial plexus injuries?**

C5 - C6.

❑❑ **In order of frequency what are the most frequently injured areas in basketball?**

Ankle, knee, foot.

❑❑ **Which organized sports are associated with an increased frequency of eye injuries and oral trauma?**

Baseball and basketball.

❑❑ **List factors associated with injury in off road bicycling.**

Excessive speed, downhill course, road obstacles, distractions, limited ability

❑❑ **T/F: Neck pain is a common complaint in cyclists because of prolonged neck extension or to transmitted forces.**

True.

❑❑ **Shin splints refer to pain in which area?**

Medial tibial.

❑❑ **What are leading causes of Medial tibial stress syndrome?**

Early season hill training and increased mileage for inexperienced runners.

❑❑ **T/F: Acute growth plate injuries are twice as common in the upper extremity as in the lower extremity in children and adolescents.**

True.

❑❑ **When should one suspect growth plate injury?**

Growth plate injury should be suspected when there is moderate or severe injury to the adjacent ligaments. Localized pain and swelling and tenderness to palpation over the site of the growth plate are a common finding hours after the injury.

❑❑ **What is the most common classification for physeal injuries?**

The Salter Harris Classification is most commonly used to classify physeal injuries. Classification is based on the radiographic findings and ranges from a non-displaced Class I to a crush type Class V injury.

❑❑ **What is the average age at onset of proximal humerus physeal stress injury (little leaguer's shoulder)?**

The proximal humerus physeal stress injury (Little Leaguer's shoulder) is a condition described in the 11 – 16 year old age group, with the average age of 14. The patient presents with gradual onset of shoulder or proximal arm pain associated with throwing.

❏❏ **What is the most common finding on examination of an adolescent with proximal humerus physeal stress injury (Little Leaguer's Shoulder)?**

The most common finding of an adolescent with this condition is tenderness to palpation over the lateral aspect of the proximal humerus.

❏❏ **What is the most common symptom in a patient presenting with Little Leaguer's Elbow?**

The most common symptom in a patient presenting with Little Leaguer's Elbow is medial elbow pain. Early in the process, patients describe relief with short periods of rest from throwing, only to recur when throwing is resumed.

❏❏ **What test may differentiate the medial elbow pain of Little Leaguer's Elbow from pure ulnar collateral ligament sprain?**

History of a valgus injury and testing the elbow in valgus stress will differentiate the medial elbow pain of Little Leaguer's elbow from pure ulnar collateral ligament sprain. The medial elbow pain from throwing may result from several foci, including medial epicondyle avulsion, microtrauma of the flexor – pronator muscle and concomitant sprain of the collateral ligament.

❏❏ **What is the most commonly reported condition in adolescents with back pain?**

Spondylosis reported in some series to account for almost 50% of low back pain in adolescents, especially gymnasts.

❏❏ **What constitutes the bony defect of spondylosis?**

The bony defect of spondylolysis occurs at the pars interarticularis (isthmic type). The defect is usually unilateral. Bilateral defects may result in spondylolysis or slippage of one vertebral body upon another.

❏❏ **What radiographic plain film is most commonly utilized to visualize the defect of spondylolysis?**

The most common radiographic view to visualize the defect of spondylolysis is the oblique spine view. In a classic lesion, the characteristic pars defect is described as the "Scotty dog" collar, with the radiolucency and sclerosis giving a collar appearance at the "neck" of the dog.

❏❏ **What is the most common cause of shoulder pain in swimmers?**

Shoulder impingement syndrome is the most common overuse injury in swimmers, and in most overhead throwing sports. Impingement occurs when the tendons of the supraspinatus, the subacromial bursa and greater tuberosity pass underneath the narrow coracoacromial arch in arm abduction and external rotation.

What is the primary pathophysiology of impingement syndrome?

The inflammation of this disorder occurs in a cycle of physical impingement leading to tendon and bursal edema and swelling, inability of the weakened cuff muscles to stabilize the humeral head, leading to increased impingement.

What are the three stages (Neer Classification) of the impingement syndrome?

The three stages of classic impingement syndrome include acute inflammation and swelling (Stage I), chronic inflammation, scar formation and tendonitis (Stage II), and rotator cuff tear (Stage III).

What are the most common contributors to overuse injury?

A significant increase in intensity, frequency and / or volume is a consistent finding in the history of the athlete presenting with an overuse injury.

What is the most important consideration in the treatment of overuse injury?

Success hinges on reduction or modification of the activity that caused the overuse injury. This common sense approach is often hindered by expectations or demands imposed on the athlete by himself, coaches or family. A team approach utilizing the physical therapist, athletic trainer, psychologist, family member and coaches is helpful in treating those difficult or progressive cases.

T/F: Decreased flexibility may contribute to an increased risk for overuse injury.

True. Injury patterns in adolescents appear to follow the flexibility pattern. Girls are usually more flexible than boys, and peak flexibility occurs at about age 14 to 15. Boys show a pattern of decreased flexibility beginning about age 7 – 8 though mid adolescence, followed by an increase in flexibility in late adolescence.

What is the weakest part of long bone in skeletally immature athletes?

The physis or growth plate is the weakest portion of long bone and more prone to injury, compared to ligament and cortical bone.

What is the most common cause of anterior knee pain in adolescents?

The most common cause of idiopathic anterior knee pain in young athletes is patellofemoral pain syndrome.

What is Osgood Schlatter disease?

Osgood Schlatter disease is a traction apophysitis affecting the insertion of the patellar tendon over the tibial tuberosity. The immature patellar tendon – tibial tubercle junction is highly susceptible to repetitive tensile stress as occurs in jumping sports.

☐☐ **What treatment would be recommended for Osgood Schlatter disease?**

A period of rest, local application of ice and flexibility exercises for the hamstrings and quadriceps muscles is helpful. This condition is usually self-limiting, but may persist for two years or longer. The athlete should be allowed to continue all sports as tolerated.

☐☐ **Identify the play positions in football that are associated with greater risk for brachial plexus injuries.**

From greatest to least, these are defensive end and linebackers, defensive lineman, offensive lineman, defensive back, offensive backs.

☐☐ **What is the most common muscle injured in soccer?**

Quadriceps muscle injury.

☐☐ **What is the most common muscle injured in football?**

Hamstrings.

☐☐ **Which phase of running is hamstring injury most likely to occur?**

Swing phase.

☐☐ **Identify three factors which contribute to the development of heat injuries.**

Increased core temperature.
Loss of body fluids.
Loss of electrolytes.

CLINICAL SPORTS MEDICINE

EVENT ADMINISTRATION

❏❏ What is the ideal interval for spacing aid stations during a running event?

2 - 2.5 miles.

❏❏ What is the duration of a suspension for any knockout in amateur boxing?

Thirty days.

❏❏ What is the duration of a suspension for a knockout in amateur boxing where loss of consciousness has occurred?

90 - 120 days.

❏❏ What degree of uncorrected vision results in an absolute prohibition from amateur boxing?

20/60 in either eye.

❏❏ What is the preferred ratio of roving emergency vehicles to participants at a mass running event?

1 vehicle: 1500 participants.

❏❏ Why are bromantan, epitestosterone, probenecid and all diuretics banned at qualifying and Olympic events?

They are all masking agents.

❏❏ What ratio of testosterone to epitestosterone is considered an " offense " at Olympic events?

6: 1 (Testosterone: epitestosterone).

❏❏ What level of urine concentration of caffeine is considered an offense at Olympic events?

>5 mcg/ml.

❑❑ **What level of urine concentration of ephedrine is considered an offense at Olympic events?**

10 mcg/ml.

❑❑ **What urine concentration of pseudoephedrine is considered an offense at Olympic events?**

>25 mcg/ml.

❑❑ **At Olympic events and qualifying events, what urine concentration of beta 2 agonists (bambuterol, clenbuterol, fenoterol, formoterol, reproterol, salbutamol, salmeterol or terbuterol) would be considered an offense?**

>1000 nanograms/ml.

❑❑ **Which hormones are considered an offense if detected at Olympic and qualifying events?**

Chorionic gonadotrophin (hCG), Pituitary or synthetic gonadotrophin (LH).

❑❑ **Which sports prohibit beta blockers?**

Shooting, archery and the biathlon.

❑❑ **What untoward effects on the male reproductive system have been reported in marijuana (THC) users?**

Decreased plasma testosterone, gynecomastia and oligospermia.

❑❑ **What is the current therapeutic use for ethanol?**

None.

❑❑ **Abuse of which hormone is associated with acromegaly?**

Human growth hormone.

❑❑ **What irreversible skeletal complication can result from anabolic steroid use?**

Closure of the epiphysis.

❑❑ **What are the effects of anabolic steroids on lipid content of the blood?**

Increase in total cholesterol, Increase in LDL, Decrease in HDL cholesterol.

❑❑ **What irreversible androgenizing effects are seen in females using anabolic steroids?**

Hirsutism, clitoromegaly and deepening of the voice.

❏❏ **What is the most commonly abused substance in the United States?**

Ethanol.

❏❏ **What is the approximate elimination time for over the counter cold preparations containing ephedrine?**

48 - 72 hours.

❏❏ **What is the approximate elimination time for fat soluble injectable steroids?**

6-12 months.

❏❏ **What is the approximate elimination time for water soluble oral anabolic steroids?**

1 - 6 weeks.

❏❏ **What is the approximate elimination time for stimulants such as amphetamines?**

1 - 7 days.

❏❏ **What is the approximate elimination time for stimulants such as cocaine in a repeated user?**

3-5 days.

❏❏ **What is the official stance of the International Olympic Committee (IOC) and the NCAA on the use of sympathomimetic vasoconstrictors such as ephedrine, phenylephrine, pseudoephedrine and tetrahydrozoline?**

All of these substances are banned.

❏❏ **What effect do anabolic steroids have on aerobic capacity?**

None.

❏❏ **Where are anabolic steroids, taken orally or injected converted to testosterone?**

Liver.

❏❏ **Which form of anabolic steroid lasts longer within the body, oral or injectable?**

Injectable.

❏❏ **What distinguishes Durabolin & Boldenone (injectable anabolic steroids) from androstenediol or other oral steroids?**

Injectable anabolic steroids do not require hepatic conversion to an active form.

❑❑ **What irreversible effect on the skeletal system can occur in skeletally immature athletes who utilize anabolic steroids ?**

Epiphyseal closure.

❑❑ **Athletes using anabolic androgenic steroids are at increase risk for the development of this hepatic lesion of blood filled cysts, with an increased tendency for traumatic rupture and hemorrhage. What are these lesions called?**

Peliosis hepatica.

❑❑ **Which beta 2 agonist, used in the treatment of asthma has been shown to have anabolic effects (i.e. promotion of protein syntheses and increased lean body mass)?**

Clenbuterol.

❑❑ **How does the use of caffeine contribute to heat related injury?**

As a diuretic it can cause dehydration leading to diminish muscular strength and endurance.

❑❑ **Within the category of stimulants, what class of drugs is considered the most potent ergogenic drug?**

Amphetamine.

❑❑ **Methylphenidate and other amphetamine derivatives have been shown to improve concentration in patients with this disorder.**

Attention deficit disorder.

❑❑ **What effect does human growth hormone have on lipid content?**

Increased serum cholesterol and increased triglycerides.

❑❑ **What effect does human growth hormone have on glucose metabolism?**

An insulin like effect which diminishes performance.

❑❑ **Athletes who elect to utilize blood doping may elevate their hematocrits above 55%. What hematologic complication do they risk by employing this technique?**

Hyperviscosity syndrome, stroke and heart failure. All of these can lead to death.

CLINICAL SPORTS MEDICINE

INJURY PREVENTION

❏❏ **What ligamentous tear has been prevented with the advent of thumb attached gloves?**

Ulnar collateral ligament of the thumb.

❏❏ **Coaches who do not allow young baseball players to throw curve pitches until they are shaving may help to prevent this syndrome.**

Little league elbow.

❏❏ **What is the recommended ratio of fluid replacement to time of intense activity?**

1 - 1.5 liters of fluid: 1 hour of intense activity.

❏❏ **What is the recommended daily allowance of calcium supplementation?**

800 mg/day.

❏❏ **Continuous passive motion is known to enhance the nutrition of what joint structure?**

Articular cartilage.

❏❏ **Utilizing two pairs of socks allows friction between socks rather than between socks and skin. This technique can prevent what common injury?**

Blisters.

❏❏ **What is the best method to prevent callus formation on the feet?**

Padding with tape or moleskin on vulnerable places on the feet.

❏❏ **What category of injury is reduced when coaches allow frequent substitutions, regular fluid breaks and shorter game times?**

Heat injuries.

❏❏ **What is the upper limit of weekly mileage to prevent overuse injuries in runners?**

30 miles.

❏❏ **Eccentrically strengthened arm extensors and posterior shoulder musculature helps to dissipate throwing forces. What overuse injury can be prevented with these steps of conditioning?**

Rotator cuff tendonitis.

❏❏ **Breakaway or low profile bases can prevent injuries to ankles, knees, hands, wrists and fingers that occur during what activity?**

Baseball slide.

❏❏ **What common steps can be taken to prevent the "yips"?**

Changing hand position.

❏❏ **What pharmacologic agents have been shown to prevent the yips?**

None.

❏❏ **Because of side to side movement, what feature must a good racquet sport shoe have that is not required for a good running shoe?**

A strong heel cup and a heel counter.

❏❏ **Age over 30, improper grip size, use of a metal racquet, average practice duration over 2 hours per day, tight strings and incorrect backhand technique (snapping wrist) are risk factors for what upper extremity overuse injury?**

Tennis elbow / Lateral epicondylitis/ strain of the extensor carpi radialis brevis.

❏❏ **What action is indicated to prevent the transmission of herpes gladiatorum from one wrestler to another?**

Isolation of infected wrestlers until the lesions are resolved.

❏❏ **What factor is most important in preventing resistance training injuries?**

Proper technique/ supervision.

❏❏ **What type of fluid is recommended for hydration for activities lasting more than one hour?**

Glucose / electrolyte solution with 6% glucose content.

❐❐   **In order to prevent heat related injuries, what simple procedure can allow coaches to monitor fluid losses in athletes?**

Supervised weigh in and weigh out procedures.

❐❐   **In order to prevent HIV exposure in treating an athlete, what three steps should health care providers take when treating any athlete with open wounds?**

Wear latex gloves when examining and managing open wounds.
Wash hands before and after treating an athlete with an open wound.
Use proper eye protection when treating open wounds.

❐❐   **What is the most important factor in preventing heat stress syndromes?**

Adequate fluid replacement.

❐❐   **Prophylactic use of which medications have been shown to prevent Raynaud's Syndrome?**

Reserpine, Prazosin (Tolazoline) and calcium channel blockers.

❐❐   **What pharmacologic options have been shown to prevent cholinergic urticaria?**

Antihistamines.

❐❐   **Which material has been shown to be most effective in the construction of safety glasses and sports eye protection?**

Polycarbonate plastic.

❐❐   **What type of protective equipment has been shown to be effective in preventing severe maxillofacial injuries in hockey players?**

Face masks.

❐❐   **What device is the most effective in the prevention of olecranon bursitis?**

Protective elbow padding.

❐❐   **Hyperextension of which structure is prevented by Duke Simpson strapping?**

Knee.

❐❐   **What type of protective equipment can prevent cervical strain (burner/ stinger)?**

Cervical collar/ support.

❏❏ **What alteration in footwear has been shown to lower the incidence of injuries in football players?**

Multiple cleated soccer style shoes.

❏❏ **What type of injury is prevented by utilizing plastic coated soccer balls (by reducing water saturation)?**

Head injuries.

❏❏ **Assuming that playing conditions are adequate, what activities are the most productive in reducing or preventing Achilles tendonitis?**

Proper warm up and stretching exercises.

❏❏ **What steps can prevent "Cauliflower ear"?**

Wearing headgear while wrestling.

❏❏ **Prohibition of what technique has resulted in significant reductions in head and neck injuries in high school football?**

Spearing.

❏❏ **Removal of which piece of equipment has resulted in significant reduction in injury rates in gymnastic competitions?**

Trampoline.

❏❏ **What is the most common musculoskeletal injury in young athletes?**

Contusions.

❏❏ **T/F: Proper stretching programs have been shown to decrease overall injury rates.**

False. No studies have documented a lower incidence of injury.

CLINICAL SPORTS MEDICINE

EMERGENCY ASSESSMENT AND TRIAGE

❑❑ **What is triage and why is it important?**

Triage refers to the rapid assessment of injured athletes and setting priorities as to the urgency of treatment and referral.

❑❑ **What is the most important step after recognition or suspicion of a cervical spine injury?**

The most important first step in cervical spine injury is insuring the airway with C spine control. Next activate the EMS system.

❑❑ **What is the current recommendation regarding football helmet removal in the case of cervical injury?**

The football helmet should be left in place unless airway management is impossible. The neck should be stabilized for transport using a spine board, cervical collar and sandbags in the prescribed manner as much as possible.

❑❑ **List two possible ways to remove the face guard in the case of cervical trauma.**

If airway management dictates removal of the faceguard, then a sharp knife can be used to cut the plastic attachments to the helmet. Alternatively, a screwdriver can be used to back out the screws attaching the face guard to the helmet. The best method is the one well thought out in advance of the injury. Be prepared and know the equipment in the pre season.

❑❑ **List four symptoms that may alert the physician to an eye emergency?**

Conditions that require immediate attention to an eye injury include blurred vision, visual field cut, sharp stabbing pain in the eye and double vision. These symptoms may be caused by a number of acute conditions and require a through history and evaluation.

❑❑ **What is the typical presentation for ear hematoma?**

Ear hematoma presents after a blow to the ear followed by throbbing pain and a fluctuant mass at the helix. The condition is most commonly seen in wrestling or rugby.

❏❏ **How can a tooth avulsion on the field be treated?**

An avulsed tooth can be rinsed in saline prior to replantation intraorally. The practitioner can transport the athlete to a definitive treatment facility with the tooth replanted if successful, or transport the tooth in saline, milk or the patient's saliva.

❏❏ **What is the treatment for acute epistaxis?**

The treatment for acute epistaxis includes covering the nasal area with a cold cloth, utilizing ice and a compressive hold on the anterior nasal region. A nasal pack is sometimes required for anterior bleeds. A posterior nasal bleed may be difficult to correct in the field setting and requires transport to a definitive treatment facility.

❏❏ **What is the recommended treatment in the field for an open fracture?**

Open fractures are treated with a sterile dressing soaked in saline or Betadine. The injured extremity is splinted without pulling exposed bone back into soft tissue, unless there is vascular compromise. Wounds caused by open fractures should not be probed in the non operative setting.

❏❏ **What is the initial treatment for traumatic amputation?**

The initial treatment after hemostatic control includes irrigation of the stump and part with saline, wrap in sterile gauze. Transport the amputated part in a plastic bag cooled on ice.

❏❏ **What is the typical presentation for anterior shoulder dislocation?**

The athlete with anterior shoulder dislocation presents after a blow to an externally rotated, abducted arm, with the painful arm abducted and internally rotated. A hollow space is palpable at the anterior deltoid, where the humeral head normally lies.

❏❏ **Under what circumstances should an athlete be transported to the nearest trauma center?**

If there is a loss of function or a life threatening situation is present.

❏❏ **T/F: When transporting an athlete on a stretcher all extremities should be in axial alignment.**

True.

❏❏ **In an adolescent or adult athlete with a suspected cervical spine injury how many team members are necessary to safely log roll the player onto a full length spine board for transport?**

Four or five.

❏❏ **What is the HOPS format for injury assessment?**

History of the injury.
Observation and inspection.
Palpation.
Special tests.

❏❏ **T/F: In the athlete who has sustained a traumatic injury, outcome is directly related to time from injury to properly delivered definitive care.**

True.

❏❏ **T/F: Standard precautions are recommended in all cases dealing with body fluids and items contaminated with body fluids.**

True. The spread of HIV is a concern as well as exposure to hepatitis from infected athletes. Immunization for Hepatitis B is also advised for medical personnel involved in emergency medical care with the above mentioned exposures.

❏❏ **What is the on field management of a ruptured globe?**

The goal in such cases is to protect the eye and transport the athlete to a definitive treatment facility with an ophthalmologic surgeon. A sterile dressing and eye protector should be applied carefully to avoid pressure against the globe. Advise the athlete not to squeeze the injured eye shut. Do not apply any topical analgesics. Do not attempt to remove clots.

❏❏ **T/F: Athletes who have sustained head trauma resulting from high energy transfer are at risk for death and should be transported immediately to a trauma center for evaluation.**

True.

❏❏ **What steps should be taken prior to considering the administration of sedation to an injured patient?**

Address the ABC's of cardiopulmonary resuscitation.
Relieve the patient's pain as much as possible (eg apply splints, etc.).
Calm & reassure athlete.

❏❏ **T/F: Injured athletes with Glasgow Coma Scales (CGS) < 14 or GCS deterioration fall into the high risk category, necessitating early transfer to a trauma facility.**

True.

❏❏ **What are the responsibilities of the referring physician in the transfer of an injured athlete?**

1. Initiate the transfer to the trauma facility.
2. Select the appropriate mode of transport and level of care required for transport.

3. Consult with the receiving physician.
4. Stabilization of the athlete's condition within the capabilities of the initial facility.
5. Transfer arrangements should not be delayed and may begin while resuscitation is ongoing.

What are the responsibilities of the receiving physician?

1. Consult about the transfer.
2. Assure that the receiving institution is qualified, able and willing to accept athlete.
3. Agree to transfer.
4. Assist the referring physician with arrangements for the appropriate mode of transport and level of care during transport or if unable to do so, assist in finding an alternate placement for the patient.

What type of information should the referring physician provide to the trauma surgeon receiving the injured athlete?

1. Identify the patient; provide pertinent data from medical history if available.
2. Provide a brief history, including prehospital data.
3. Initial findings, therapy given and response to therapy.

What is " spinal shock "?

Spinal shock refers to the flaccidity and loss of reflexes after spinal cord injury.

What is the appropriate method to remove a football helmet if attempts to remove the helmet result in pain and paraesthesia?

Remove helmet with a cast cutter.

T/F: In head injured patients, hypotonic fluids should not be used in fluid resuscitation.

True.

Identify signs and symptoms that would alert you to the possibility of pelvic fracture?

1. Ecchymosis over the iliac wings, pubis, labia or scrotum.
2. Pain on palpation of the pelvic ring.
3. Mobility of the pelvis in response to gentle anterior to posterior pressure with the heels of the hands on both anterior iliac spines and the symphysis pubis.

T/F: Cardiovascular dynamics are altered in athletes who have rigorous training routines.

True. Blood volume, cardiac output and stroke volume can be increased; resting pulse is lower than in non athletes. Therefore the usual responses to hypovolemia may not be manifest, even though significant blood loss has occurred.

❏❏ **T/F: Athletes who have ingested alcohol prior to exercise are at increased risk of hypothermia because of the associated vasodilation.**

True.

❏❏ **What is the initial on field management of an open pneumothorax?**

Prompt closing of the defect with a sterile occlusive dressing, large enough to overlap the wound's edges. Tape on three sides allowing a flutter type valve effect to occur. As soon as possible a chest tube should be placed remote from the wound and the initial dressing taped securely on all four sides. The patient should be transported to a trauma facility as soon as possible.

❏❏ **How would you identify a tension pneumothorax?**

Chest pain, air hunger, respiratory distress, tachycardia, hypotension.
Tracheal deviation, unilateral absence of breath sounds.
Neck vein distention.
Cyanosis as a late manifestation.

❏❏ **T/F: Radiologic confirmation is required prior to intervention for a tension pneumothorax.**

False. Tension pneumothorax is a clinical diagnosis. It would be inappropriate to delay intervention awaiting radiologic evaluation.

❏❏ **What is the on field treatment for a tension pneumothorax?**

Immediate decompression.

❏❏ **What is commotio cordis?**

A lethal ventricular dysrhythmia occurring following a direct blow to the precordium during an "electrically vulnerable" period.

❏❏ **What is the recommended treatment for commotio cordis?**

Defibrillation.
CPR.

❏❏ **Under what conditions would you consider allowing a football player to return to competition following a burner?**

All symptoms must have subsided.
Strength must have returned to normal.
Full, painless range of motion of the neck must be demonstrated.

❏❏ **What is the most common cause of traumatic death in youth baseball players?**

Commotio cordis is the single most common cause of traumatic death in youth baseball players. In this condition, the heart suffers a structural, nonfunctional injury and subsequent dysrhythmia from the blunt force of the baseball striking the sternum. Several case reports of fatal commotio cordis from not only baseball, but also softball and hockey pucks are documented in the medical literature.

❏❏ T/F: Traumatic subluxation of the hip can result in avascular necrosis and osteonecrosis of the femoral head.

True. Although avascular necrosis of the femoral head is classically reported in hip dislocation, the interruption of blood supply is possible with subluxation of the femoral head.

❏❏ What is the equipment most implicated as the main contributor to wrist injury in male gymnastics?

The pommel horse has been implicated as the main contributor to wrist injury in male gymnastics. The wrist is subjected to the high intensity of impact and the stress of repetition.

❏❏ What is the most important consideration when approaching the unconscious athlete on the field?

The health care leader must make certain that no additional injury occurs through unnecessary motion of the head and neck. The first priority is to stabilize the head and neck in neutral position.

❏❏ What radiographic views are required to clear the cervical spine of bony injury?

The minimum radiographic views to clear the cervical spine of bony injury include the anteroposterior view, the lateral view to include C7 – T1 and the open mouth odontoid view.

❏❏ What is the minimum equipment necessary to perform an eye examination in the acutely injured eye?

The minimum equipment necessary to perform an eye examination is the vision card, penlight, sterile fluorescein strips, sterile eye pads, eye shields, tape, sterile cotton tipped swabs and sterile irrigating solution.

❏❏ What is hyphema?

Hyphema is a collection of free blood in the anterior chamber of the eye. It is the most common intraocular injury associated with sports. Initially, hyphema may appear as a haze in the anterior chamber.

❏❏ What is the most common carpal bone to be fractured?

The scaphoid is the most common carpal bone to be fractured. Wrist pain after a fall onto an outstretched hand is a scaphoid fracture until proven otherwise.

☐☐ **Why is avulsion of the flexor digitorum profundus a surgical urgency?**

Avulsion of the flexor digitorum profundus, or Jersey finger, occurs when the Distal interphalangeal (DIP) joint is forcibly extended while the flexor digitorum profundus is acutely contracted. The tendon can then retract to the level of the palm, the PIP joint or the AI pulley. In the absence of surgical intervention, the blood supply and joint function is compromised. In the case of tendon retraction to the palm, surgical intervention is required within 7 – 10 days.

☐☐ **Describe the reduction of a patellar dislocation.**

The patella dislocates laterally in response to lateral forces caused by external rotation of the tibia relative to the femur. The patella is reduced by bringing the leg into extension, while applying gentle medial pressure to the patella. The knee is then immobilized in extension for two to four weeks.

☐☐ **Describe the mechanism of a posterior dislocation of the knee in sports?**

The posterior dislocation of the knee results from a direct blow to the anterior, proximal tibia, driving it posteriorly. This most commonly occurs in football, as the helmet strikes the tibia of a knee in full extension. This condition is an orthopedic emergency, as the popliteal artery may be stretched or torn.

☐☐ **What are the classic signs of tension pneumothorax?**

The classic signs of tension pneumothorax include absent or diminished breath sounds, tracheal shift to the opposite side and hypotension.

☐☐ **What is the emergency treatment for tension pneumothorax?**

The on field emergency treatment for tension pneumothorax is placement of a 14 gauge catheter into the second intercostal space, at the midclavicular line.

CLINICAL SPORTS MEDICINE

DIAGNOSIS AND TREATMENT OF ACUTE MUSCULOSKELETAL INJURIES

❑❑ **List the most common stress fracture site for the following sports: javelin, ballet dancing, fencing, skating.**

Javelin throwing - ulnar olecranon.
Ballet dancing – tibia.
Fencing – pubis.
Skating – fibula.

❑❑ **What is the differential diagnosis for stress fractures in children?**

Infection.
Malignancy.
Osteoid osteoma.

❑❑ **What is the most frequently strained muscle?**

The " hamstrings". In sprinters as many as 50% can suffer strains during the course of their careers.

❑❑ **A football player, previously diagnosed with turf toe comes to you after practice with complaint of continued pain and swelling over the medial plantar aspect of his great toe. You x ray his foot and note a bipartite sesamoid bone. What can cause sesamoid pain?**

Bursitis, stress fracture, chondromalacia, contusion/crush fracture, osteochondritis, sesamoiditis in association with collagen vascular disease.

❑❑ **What is the differential diagnosis for the above patient?**

Gout, tarsal tunnel syndrome, flexor hallices longus tendonitis, osteoarthritis of MTP joint, synovitis of MTP joint, rheumatoid arthritis.

❑❑ **What is Iselin's Disease?**

Traction apophysitis of the base of the fifth metatarsal. It is commonly seen in prepubertal children engaged in running and jumping sports that place stress on the forefoot.

❐❐ **What is the treatment of plantar fasciitis?**

Initial rest, NSAIDS, Achilles tendon stretch, physical therapy.

❐❐ **Where are clavicular fractures most likely to occur?**

Eighty percent of clavicular fractures occur in the shaft of the bone; 15% distally and 5% medially. Lateral fractures can be further subclassified into type I (intact ligament and minimal displaced fracture), type II (detached ligaments with fracture displacement) and type III (fracture of the articular surface).

❐❐ **What structural abnormalities predispose to impingement syndrome?**

Subacromial space calcium deposits.
Acromioclavicular spurring.
Thickened coracoacromial ligament.
Type 3 curved or Type 3 hooked acromion.

❐❐ **What is the Hawkins and Kennedy test (Speed's test)?**

Used to aid in the diagnosis of biceps tendonitis, the athlete attempts forward flexion of the shoulder joint with the elbow extended and the forearm supinated. Resistance to this motion causes pain in the bicipital groove when tendon inflammation is present.

❐❐ **What X ray studies are most helpful in demonstrating acromioclavicular deformities and acromial spurs?**

AP, 30 degree caudal tilt.
Scapular outlet view (lateral 10 degree caudal tilt).

❐❐ **What physical exam findings are associated with glenoid labral tear?**

Diffuse shoulder pain catching and a clicking or popping sensation. These symptoms are caused by a labral flap blocking glenohumeral articulation. It is usually associated with glenohumeral instability.

❐❐ **What risk factors are associated with the development of heel spurs in athletes?**

1. 75% association with plantar fasciitis.
2. May be associated with systemic disease - Reiter's Syndrome, ankylosing spondylitis, gout, rheumatoid arthritis.
3. Most commonly are the result of traction at the heel.
4. 10 - 30 % asymptomatic.

❐❐ **Which physical examination findings help the clinician to distinguish between Soleus and Gastrocnemius spasm?**

With the knee in flexion, a tight Soleus muscle should restrict dorsal flexion of the foot. With the knee extended, the gastrocnemius muscle is tightened and exerts a limiting force on foot.

❏❏ **What risk factors are associated with the development of Achilles tendonitis in athletes?**

Inflexibility of the Achilles tendon muscle complex.
A recent increase in exercise.
A recent change in shoeware.
Foot over pronation.

❏❏ **What age group is most commonly at risk for Achilles' tendon rupture and what physical findings are present with this diagnosis?**

Age 30 - 50. Weak ankle flexion and a palpable tendon defect along with a positive Thompson's test. No demonstrable plantar flexion of the foot upon squeezing of the calf muscle.

❏❏ **What is the position of healing (immobilization and splinting) of the following fractures: metacarpal, MCP, DIP/PIP ?**

Metacarpal – neutral.
MCP - 30 degrees flexion.
DIP/PIP - 30 degrees flexion.

❏❏ **T/F: After suffering a dislocation of the third PIP joint a basketball player has an X ray taken which reveals a 20% nondisplaced avulsion fracture of the articular surface. Surgical repair of this lesion is required.**

False. Phalangeal fractures with volar displacement of the fracture chip or involvement of greater than 25 - 30% of the articular surface should be referred to a hand surgeon for possible operative repair.

❏❏ **What is a boutonniere deformity of the finger and how does it differ from a pseudoboutonnière deformity?**

A boutonniere deformity is the rupture of the central slip of the extensor digitorum commons muscle as it crosses over the PIP joint. The patient is able to flex the distal joint, which is not the case in a pseudo boutonniere deformity.

❏❏ **What pneumonic is useful in remembering the treatment course for shoulder dislocations?**

T Traumatic shoulder instability.
U Unilateral injury.
B Bankart lesion.
S Surgical management.

❏❏ **A football player attempts to tackle an opposing player by grabbing the opponent. After the play he runs to the sidelines complaining of severe finger pain and inability to flex the third PIP joint. What is the diagnosis?**

Avulsion of the flexor digitorum profundus tendon or "Jersey finger". Treatment requires surgical tendon reattachment after initial X ray and splinting.

❑❑ **What is a Steiner's lesion?**

Seen in gamekeeper or skier's thumb, it is the entrapment of the adductor aponeurosis between the torn ends of the thumb's ulnar collateral ligament. When evaluating this injury the thumb MCP joint must be stressed gently in extension and in slight flexion to insure ligament integrity. An X ray should be taken to rule out bony avulsion or intra articular fracture.

❑❑ **What injury represents 60% of the upper extremity injuries that are associated with skiers?**

Ulnar collateral ligament injury (Gamekeeper's or Skier's thumb).

❑❑ **What degree of angulation is abnormal when stress testing the MCP joint in a skier's thumb injury?**

Greater than 35 degrees signifies a complete tear of the ulnar collateral ligament, requiring surgical repair.

❑❑ **What percentage of scaphoid fractures involve the proximal portion?**

20%. This is significant because the blood supply in 30 % of patients is mainly from the distal pole making proximal fractures prone to avascular necrosis. Seventy percent of scaphoid fractures are located midbone.

❑❑ **T/F: Transverse fractures of the base of the first metacarpal (Bennett's fracture) requires percutaneous pin fixation to maintain reasonable bony alignment.**

False. Only fractures entering the joint (Rolando fractures) may require fixation. Treatment options depend on the degree of fracture displacement and commutation.

❑❑ **What X ray view best demonstrates Hill Sach lesion of the posterior lateral humeral head?**

AP internal rotation, Stryker notch view.

❑❑ **What is the most common complication of anterior shoulder dislocation?**

Recurrent dislocation is the most common complication following acute traumatic anterior shoulder dislocation.

❑❑ **What percentage of shoulder dislocations are traumatic?**

95%.

❑❑ **What is a Bankart lesion?**

A Bankart lesion is a detachment of the glenoid labrum and capsule from the anterior glenoid rim. A small bony fragment from the glenoid rim may also be present.

❏❏ **What is the leading cause of permanent elbow disability?**

Osteochondritis dissecans.

❏❏ **Which tennis players are most likely at risk for developing lateral epicondylitis?**

Novice players, players over 35, players engaged in multiple games per week.

❏❏ **Which shoulder injury is present with a positive drop test?**

Rotator cuff tear.

❏❏ **What is the most common shoulder injury in throwing sport athletes?**

Supraspinatus tendinitis.

❏❏ **A baseball pitcher presents with acute shoulder pain. In this scenario what is the most common acute shoulder injury?**

Rotator cuff injury. High risk sports include swimming, weight lifting, volleyball and all throwing sports.

❏❏ **A nationally ranked medley swimmer presented to you with complaints of shoulder pain. Which stroke is most likely the cause of his impingement syndrome?**

The Butterfly stroke.

❏❏ **What is Freiberg's test?**

Forced internal rotation of the hip with the patient in a prone position. A positive test is suggestive of piriformis syndrome.

❏❏ **What is a hip pointer?**

A contusion of the iliac crest characterized by sudden local severe pain. Occasionally an audible pop or snap is noted. Local swelling and burning can be extensive due to the localized hemorrhage. Radiographs are indicated in order to rule out an associated fracture.

❏❏ **T/F: Shoulder pain without apprehension in external rotation, extension and abduction is consistent with shoulder instability.**

False. Shoulder instability is associated with a positive apprehension test.

❏❏ **T/F: There is a six fold greater rate of recurrent injury in ACL deficient knee skiers than in uninjured high level skiers.**

True.

❑❑ **A bicyclist comes to you with complaints of weakness of finger adduction and numbness of the fourth and fifth fingers. What is the most likely diagnosis and how would you treat it?**

Ulnar neuritis (bicyclist palsy). It is treated with rest, adjustment of bicycle handlebars and use of padded grips/gloves. NSAIDS and a rehab exercise program can help relieve persistent symptoms.

❑❑ **Volkmann's ischemic contracture is associated with what acute injury in children? What physical findings are associated with this lesion?**

Supracondylar fracture of the humerus. Compartmental ischemia may result in flexor muscle scarring and contracture along with ulnar and median nerve paralysis.

❑❑ **A 15-year-old skate boarder presents to you with a Monteggia fracture of the ulna? What critical associated injury needs to be considered?**

A Monteggia fracture involves the proximal 1/3 of the ulna and is often associated with dislocation of the radial head.

❑❑ **What is Panner's disease?**

Panner's disease is osteochondritis of the capitellum secondary to aseptic or avascular necrosis. Ninety percent of cases occur in males with 95% unilateral involvement in the dominant arm. It commonly occurs before the age of 9 but can present later.

❑❑ **T/F: MRI is the " gold standard" for acute cervical spine injury.**

False. CT scanning remains the gold standard for acute neck trauma. No single form of imaging accurately visualizes both hard and soft tissue abnormalities. MRI remains the study of choice for evaluating suspected spinal cord injuries, occult vascular injuries, disc herniation and ligament tears.

❑❑ **T/F: A pre exercise stretching program is essential in preventing acute athletic injuries.**

False. Despite its place in general sports culture, pre exercise stretching programs have not been shown to significantly reduce the risk of exercise related injury.

❑❑ **The major cause of major spinal injury in hockey is the result of getting hit in the head or neck with a hockey stick.**

False. Sixty five percent of major spinal injuries were the result of the injured player being checked from behind and pushed into the boards.

❑❑ **What is the treatment of medial epicondylitis?**

Prevention of progression of symptoms by reduction of elbow stress.
Acute relief of symptoms with ice, rest, ultrasound and other modalities.
Gradual isometric arm exercise to the point of pain tolerance.
ROM and isometric exercise of the shoulder and wrist.

Gradual progression of throwing with increasing velocity and distance.

❏❏ **A baseball pitcher presents with complaints of pain, swelling, popping and locking sensation in his throwing elbow. What phases of throwing are most likely to be responsible for his symptoms?**

The cocking and acceleration phases of throwing place great valgus stress on the lateral elbow joint, predisposing to osteochondritis dissecans and the subsequent symptoms.

❏❏ **A tennis player presents with complaints of elbow pain. What provocative tests are most likely to be positive?**

Lateral epicondylitis is most common in tennis players. Any test which stresses the extensor group of muscles, originating from the lateral epicondyle is likely to be positive, i.e. resistance to wrist extension, resistance to extension of the elbow with the wrist flexed and the forearm pronated and resistance to third finger extension.

❏❏ **A rugby player, after receiving a severe contusion to his upper arm complains of difficulty with flexion and supination. What nerve and muscle are most likely involved?**

The musculocutaneous nerve innervates the biceps brachii, which is an elbow flexor and forearm supinator.

❏❏ **What muscle is most likely involved in tennis elbow (lateral epicondylitis)?**

Extensor carpi radialis brevis is directly attached to the lateral epicondyle. Microtears and tendon strains occur just distal to the bone tendon junction.

❏❏ **T/F: Stress fractures are more common among college freshman and sophomore college athletes than junior and senior athletes.**

True.

❏❏ **What is the most common fracture of the proximal humerus seen in adolescence?**

Salter - Harris type II fracture because the physis of the proximal humerus is one of the last to close.

❏❏ **What external forces are most likely to result in acromioclavicular joint dislocation?**

Blows to the posterior aspect of the acromion and scapular spine.

❏❏ **A wrestler presents with a positive Finkelstein test (pain over the lateral dorsal wrist with the patient's flexed thumb placed inside the flexed fingers and the wrist deviated to the ulnar side). What is the most likely diagnosis? Which tendon or tendons are involved?**

DeQuervain's tendonitis involving the extensor pollicus brevis and adductor pollicus longus.

❏❏ **A 30-year-old runner has a dull ache in the mid buttocks associated with prolonged sitting and walking up inclines. Signs and symptoms are decreased or absent when lying supine. What is the most likely diagnosis? What is the differential diagnosis?**

Piriformis syndrome. The differential diagnosis includes SI joint dysfunction, ischial bursitis, coccydynia, spinal tumors/ stenosis and facet syndrome.

❏❏ **A weightlifter complains of increasing hand/wrist pain, morning stiffness and difficulty opposing his thumb to his fifth finger. Which additional tests would help to confirm the diagnosis?**

This patient has symptoms consistent with carpal tunnel syndrome.

1. Phalen's (wrist flexion) test - numbness with opposing hands placed fully flexed against one another.
2. Tourniquet test - Inflating blood pressure cuff higher than the patient's systolic blood pressure and causing hand numbness in the medial nerve innervation
3. Medial nerve percussion (Tinel test) - pain elicited by tapping the center of the carpal tunnel
4. Medial nerve compression test - numbness after 15 - 120 seconds of direct pressure on the carpal tunnel

❏❏ **What anatomic structure passes through the tunnel of Gugon (pisiform hamate tunnel)?**

The ulnar nerve and artery.

❏❏ **A rower presents after several weeks of heavy practice with flexion weakness of the distal thumb and fingers. On physical exam you note an abnormal OK sign - the patient is not able to flex the inter phalangeal joint of the thumb. What is the diagnosis?**

Anterior interosseous nerve palsy. The nerve is a branch of the medial nerve injured by repetitive heavy exercise of the forearm.

❏❏ **An inline skater without wrist pads falls backwards with arms outstretched. In addition to lateral dorsal wrist pain, there is maximum tenderness in the anatomical snuffbox. With initial X rays negative, what is the initial treatment approach?**

The history and exam are consistent with a probable scaphoid fracture. A thumb spica cast should be applied for 10 - 14 days. If repeat X rays are positive a long arm cast is applied for two weeks followed by 6 - 8 weeks of a short arm cast until clinical and radiographic healing has occurred. Bone scan and CT can be helpful with the initial fracture diagnosis.

❏❏ **A female soccer player is complaining of medial thigh pain radiating into the inguinal region. The physical exam demonstrates increased pain with stretching of the groin muscles and localized pelvic pain. What is the most likely cause?**

Osteitis pubis (gracilis syndrome) - an inflammation of the pubic symphysis. It is common in soccer, track, baseball and ice hockey players.

❏❏ **A long jumper exhibits signs of weakness with hip abduction, gluteal atrophy, a deep ache with palpation and a Trendelenburg gait. Assuming no sciatic nerve involvement, what is the most likely cause?**

Superior gluteal nerve entrapment.

❏❏ **Name the triad of stress fracture sites occur in distance runners.**

Pelvis, femur and sacrum.

❏❏ **T/F: Facial bone fracture in skiers most commonly result from being struck by their own equipment.**

False. While dentoalveolar trauma is likely to result from skiers hitting their own equipment, facial bone fractures are usually caused by collision with other people or stationary objects on the slopes.

❏❏ **What is a Hill Sach lesion?**

A Hill Sach lesion is a compression fracture of the posterior lateral articulation surface of the humeral head. It is present over 2/3 of recurrent dislocation cases.

❏❏ **What are the two most common sites of stress fractures in athletes?**

The tibia and the metatarsals. The tibia is the more common of the two sites.

❏❏ **T/F: An ACL tear in young female soccer players is an important risk factor for developing early radiographic signs of arthritis.**

True. In a recent study 1/3 of competitive female soccer players developed radiographic arthritic changes within 12 years of ACL repair.

❏❏ **Of the following risk factors for developing stress fractures, which is the most important factor in track athletes: biomechanical failure, disordered eating, low bone density or prior history of stress fracture?**

Low bone density.

❏❏ **What is the differential diagnosis of a tibial stress fracture?**

Medial tibial stress syndrome, Shin splints, popliteal artery entrapment syndrome and exertional compartment syndrome.

❏❏ A 21-year-old collegiate track athlete presents to you complaining of lateral ankle pain. This began yesterday when she collided with another runner, "twisted" her ankle and heard a "pop". She states she could not continue the workouts and has been limping very badly since. Physical examination reveals moderate swelling and ecchymosis. During weight bearing and ambulation she has considerable pain. She is tender over the involved structures. Her anterior draw test is positive with significant excursion. In addition, her inversion stress test has a very soft end point. Her compression test does not reproduce any pain. According to the history and physical examination, how would you grade her sprain?

Grade II.

❏❏ According to the above history and physical examination, name the ligaments that are injured.

Anterior talofibular and Calcaneofibular.

❏❏ In the same patient, we described a negative compression test. This confirms the integrity of what structure?

Syndesmosis.

❏❏ The Ottawa ankle rules can be used to determine when radiographic studies are indicated. What is the most common physical finding, which indicates the need for radiologic examination?

Bony tenderness.

❏❏ A 34-year-old runner presents to your office once again for complaints consistent with the diagnosis of plantar fasciitis. You have seen him on at least two other occasions in the past for the same thing. However, you do realize that he is an "obsessed" runner who doesn't like to stop running. You feel confident of your diagnosis because he manifests the classic signs of plantar fasciitis. Describe the "classic" sign.

Heel pain that is worse with the first few steps in the morning.

❏❏ On examination of this same patient, you note that he has pain on palpation quite typical of this diagnosis. Where do you expect the point of maximal tenderness of the calcaneus to be located?

Anteromedially.

❏❏ T/F: Nail bed lacerations associated with large subungual hematomas require nail removal and suture of the nail bed when they involve 50% or more of the nail.

True.

❏❏ **Describe what is meant by a "mallet" finger.**

A mallet finger is a flexion deformity of the distal interphalangeal joint caused by disruption of the extensor mechanism.

❏❏ **A collegiate football player presents to you on the sideline of a football practice. He is complaining of tenderness along the volar aspect of his right finger. He indicates swelling and tenderness along the volar aspect of the distal interphalangeal joint (DIP). Flexion of the proximal interphalangeal joint (PIP) and MP joints are preserved however he is unable to flex the DIP joint. Radiographs reveal a "fleck" of bone from the volar aspect of the distal phalanx. What is the appropriate management of this injury?**

Splinting, ice, referral to an orthopedist or hand surgeon.

CLINICAL SPORTS MEDICINE

CHRONIC MEDICAL PROBLEMS IN THE ATHLETE

❏❏ What is the most common cause of sudden death in athletes greater than age 35 years?

Coronary artery disease.

❏❏ What is the most prevalent risk factor for coronary artery disease?

Sedentary life style.

❏❏ What is the most common cardiac abnormality in Marfan's Syndrome?

Mitral Valve Prolapse.

❏❏ According to the 26th Bethesda Conference what time period of convalescence is required for an athlete with myocarditis?

Six months.

❏❏ What criteria must be met before an athlete may return to competition after suffering from myocarditis?

Normal ventricular function.
Normal cardiac dimensions.
No clinically relevant arrhythmias on ambulatory monitoring.

❏❏ What is the most common cause of myocarditis in the United States?

Coxsackievirus B.

❏❏ What is the most common cause of sudden death in athletes less than age 35 years?

Hypertrophic cardiomyopathy.

❏❏ List common auscultative findings indicative of cardiac pathology in an athlete.

1. Diastolic murmurs.
2. Systolic murmurs at the lower sternal border, augmented by Valsalva maneuver and decrease with squatting.

❏❏ **Which of the following electrocardiographic changes are consistent with the "Athletic Heart Syndrome"?**

Downsloping ST segment depression.
Third degree heart block.
Prolonged QT$_c$ interval.
Left ventricular hypertrophy by voltage criteria.
Septal Q waves.
T wave inversion that normalizes with exercise.

❏❏ **What period of detraining is required for the electrocardiographic changes of the "athletic heart syndrome "to revert to normal?**

Eight weeks.

❏❏ **In athletes over age 30 years what percentage suffered death from coronary artery disease?**

73% - 95% in published studies.

❏❏ **What is the most common cause of iron deficiency anemia among female distance runners?**

Menstrual loss.

❏❏ **What is the most common nutritional deficiency in athletes?**

Iron deficiency with or without anemia.

❏❏ **What are common symptoms of anemia in athletes?**

Fatigue, dyspnea with exertion, decrease in performance.

❏❏ **What are common signs of anemia in athletes?**

Pale conjunctiva, pale skin and nail beds, orthostatic changes.

❏❏ **What is "sports anemia" or " athletic pseudoanemia"?**

A normal physiological response to strenuous exercise is an increase in plasma volume (due to immediate decrease in plasma volume with compensatory volume increase secondary to activation of renin, aldosterone and vasopressin) without a change in red call mass. This dilutional anemia is normal and requires no treatment.

❏❏ **What is "foot strike" hemolysis?**

Although attributed to intravascular hemolysis secondary to the foot striking the ground in runners, it has been described in swimmers, rowers and weight lifters. Theories include (1) temperature effects from exercise (2) destruction of older red blood cells with exercise and (3) increased fragility of red blood cells with exercise.

❏❏ **How is "foot strike" hemolysis treated?**

It is rarely a clinically relevant anemia and usually requires no treatment.

❏❏ **How is iron deficiency diagnosed in the adult athlete?**

Low hemoglobin (< 13.5 g/dl), low hematocrit, low mean corpuscular volume, hypochromic red blood cells, low serum ferritin level (< 20 micrograms/ liter) and decreased percentage of serum iron.

❏❏ **What is the most common hereditary hematologic disease in athletes?**

Sickle cell disease.

❏❏ **What effect does sickle cell trait have on exercise?**

None.

❏❏ **What problems can occur in athletes with sickle cell disease?**

Vascular occlusion and infarct, infection, and rhabdomyolysis are the major complications. Avoid dehydration, temperature increases or altitude changes to prevent vascular occlusion. Athletes should receive the pneumococcal vaccine. Prophylactic penicillin is indicated in those post splenectomy. Folate supplementation is recommended.

❏❏ **What are "indicator" diseases for acquired immunodeficiency syndrome (AIDS) in adults?**

Herpes bronchitis, Kaposi's sarcoma, Pneumocystis carinii infection, cytomegalovirus infection.

❏❏ **When do most splenic rupture occur during acute mononucleosis?**

Between day 4 and 21 of the illness.

❏❏ **List three reasons why athletes should not exercise with a fever above 100.4 degrees Fahrenheit?**

Poor thermoregulatory function.
Increased theoretical risk of specific viral myocarditis infections if exercise during viremia.
Poor athletic performance may predispose athlete to other injuries such as slower response time, poor concentration

❏❏ **What are the major causes of pneumonia in young athletes?**

Viral, Mycoplasma pneumoniae, Streptococcus pneumoniae.

❏❏ **When may an athlete with pneumonia return to play?**

When the athlete is volume replete, afebrile, asymptomatic (no cough or shortness of breath). Many athletes demonstrate bronchospasm with exercise following pneumonia and require treatment during the recovery period.

❏❏ **What is the major bacterial pathogen responsible for otitis externa in athletes?**

Pseudomonas aeruginosa.

❏❏ **When may an athlete with otitis externa return to play?**

When otalgia and balance problems have resolved.

❏❏ **How is human immunodeficiency virus (HIV) disease transmitted among athletes?**

Similar to the general population HIV is transmitted via unprotected sexual activities, needle borne blood transmission, blood or blood products transmission, and transmission of infected blood into wounds or mucous membranes.

❏❏ **What is the risk of transmission between athletes in sports?**

Very low. Only one case reported in the literature and not well documented. Urine, sweat and tears have NOT been implicated in the transmission of the human immunodeficiency virus.

❏❏ **Which sports prohibit HIV infected athletes from competition?**

State boxing organizations have required HIV testing and ban HIV positive athletes from competition.

❏❏ **What is the "neck check" principle in allowing athletes to return to practice or competition with infectious symptoms?**

If the symptoms are above the neck (headache, rhinorrhea, stuffy nose, sore throat, ear ache), the athlete may return to play if there is no fever. If the symptoms are below the neck (cough, chest pain, abdominal pain, vomiting, diarrhea, myalgia, weakness, shortness of breath, malaise) then the athlete should NOT return to play until these symptoms have resolved. (There is theoretical evidence that exercise during viremia predisposes the athlete to myocarditis and its sequelae.)

❏❏ **When may an athlete with streptococcal pharyngitis return to play?**

The athlete should be afebrile and started on antibiotics for 24 hours.

❏❏ **What is the incubation period for infectious mononucleosis (Ebstein Barr Virus)?**

30 - 50 days. This may make exposure confirmation difficult.

❏❏ **What is the prodrome of infectious mononucleosis?**

The prodrome consists of malaise, fatigue, myalgias, headache and poor appetite and generally lasts 3 - 5 days.

❏❏ **What are the classic signs of infectious mononucleosis?**

Sore throat with tonsillar hypertrophy (exudate occurs in 1/3; concurrent streptococcal pharyngitis occurs in 5 - 30 %), enlarged anterior and posterior lymph nodes, fever, palatine petechiae, morbilliform skin exanthem. Symptoms may be quite variable and infectious mononucleosis has been termed the "Great Impersonator".

❏❏ **What are the complications of infectious mononucleosis?**

Airway obstruction due to hypertrophy of the adenoids and tonsillar tissue, ruptured spleen (0.1 - 0.2 %), concurrent streptococcal pharyngitis, hepatitis, encephalitis, Guillain Barré syndrome, less compliant brain tissue predisposing to increased risk from head trauma.

❏❏ **A 10-year-old swimmer is brought to the office complaining of otalgia and otorrhea. The pain has been gradually increasing over the last several days beginning after his last swim meet. He also complains of a loss of hearing and a feeling of fullness. There is no history of fever, chills or upper respiratory tract infection. Your examination is impaired, as you are unable to visualize the tympanic membrane due to swelling and debris. What is your most appropriate next step?**

Gentle insertion of a cotton wick with instillation of topical medication.

❏❏ **What is the most common precipitant of this disorder?**

Excessive moisture.

❏❏ **What are the medical benefits of exercise for the athlete with type II diabetes?**

Increased insulin sensitivity.
Improved long term glucose control.
Improved lipid profile.
Improved weight control.
Decreased risk for cardiovascular disease.

❏❏ **What are the medical benefits of exercise for the athlete with type I diabetes?**

Improved lipid profile.
Decreased risk for cardiovascular disease.
Improved peer acceptance in adolescent groups.

❏❏ **T/F: Long term studies have NOT confirmed improved long term glucose control in type I diabetics.**

True.

❑❑ **What is the "ideal" glucose range for athletes with type I diabetes beginning an endurance event?**

Most athletes perform best in the range of 120 - 180 mg/dl.

❑❑ **How do you define hypertension for an adolescent athlete?**

$\geq$ 136/86.

❑❑ **List nonpharmacologic methods for treating hypertension.**

Regular aerobic exercise, weight loss, dietary sodium restriction, increased potassium dietary intake, increased calcium dietary intake, reduction of alcohol intake, relaxation techniques (meditation, biofeedback, massage, muscle relaxation).

❑❑ **What are the benefits of exercise for the hypertensive athlete?**

Enhanced weight loss, lower systolic and diastolic blood pressure, improved fitness and lower mortality risk.

❑❑ **What are the acute effects of aerobic exercise in hypertensive athletes?**

Exercise elevates stroke volume via increases in stroke volume, heart rate, cardiac contractility and vascular resistance. The net effect is a transient increase in systolic and diastolic blood pressure.

❑❑ **According to the 26th Bethesda Conference guidelines, what is the treatment goal of adult athletes with mild to moderate hypertension for participation in dynamic exercise?**

140/90.

❑❑ **How common is exercise induced asthma / bronchospasm in athletes?**

Exercise induced asthma occurs in 10 % of all athletes. It is higher in those with allergic rhinitis (50%) and baseline asthma (90%).

❑❑ **In addition to exercise list other precipitating factors for exercise induced bronchospasm?**

Cold air, environmental pollutants, viruses, allergens, smoke.

❑❑ **Which sports are more likely to be associated with exercise induced bronchospasm?**

Running outdoors (cross country, soccer, rugby), cross country skiing, ice hockey, cross country cycling, basketball.

❑❑ **Which sports are least likely to produce exercise induced bronchospasm?**

Swimming, sprint running, indoor sports with regulated temperature and humidity.

❏❏ **List common symptoms of exercise induced asthma/ bronchospasm?**

Cough, shortness of breath, chest pain, tightness, variable or poor performance, cough following exercise ("locker room" cough) and in young athletes abdominal pain may also be reported.

❏❏ **How is exercise induced bronchospasm diagnosed?**

A decrease of $\geq 15\%$ in FEV_1 with exercise

❏❏ **What is the refractory period?**

A period of time following a short bout of exercise during which exercise induced bronchospasm is diminished. This period may last up to four hours and is considered secondary to prostaglandin release.

❏❏ **What is the late phase response?**

This refers to bronchospasm occurring 4 - 12 hours following exercise. Debated theories include either baseline asthma under poor control or a specific late response to exercise.

❏❏ **What are some of the non pharmacologic methods for treating exercise induced bronchospasm?**

Training and conditioning.
Appropriate choice of activity.
Proper warm up and cool downs.
Face masks, mufflers.
Environmental modification.

❏❏ **When do symptoms of exercise induced bronchospasm typically occur?**

6-20 minutes after strenuous exercise.

❏❏ **List common foods associated with exercise induced anaphylaxis in susceptible individuals?**

Celery, nuts, shellfish, wine, tomatoes, strawberry and peach.

❏❏ **How soon after ingestion of specific foods in these athletes does exercise induced anaphylaxis occur?**

Exercise within four hours after ingestion of specific foods in susceptible individuals may produce symptoms.

❏❏ **Can aspirin ingestion affect the occurrence of exercise induced anaphylaxis?**

Yes. Specific food and aspirin ingestion together with exercise increases the likelihood of occurrence.

❏❏ **Which forms of exercise have been associated with anaphylaxis?**

Jogging, aerobics, brisk walking, racquet sports, cycling, swimming and skiing.

❏❏ **What are the typical signs of exercise induced anaphylaxis?**

Fatigue, urticaria, angioedema, laryngospasm, respiratory distress, nausea and vomiting.

❏❏ **What are some of the non pharmacologic methods for exercise induced anaphylaxis?**

1. Avoid exercising within four (4) hours of eating.
2. Avoid exercising outdoors during pollen allergy season (for those who are pollen sensitive).
3. Avoid exercising during menses in susceptible young women.
4. Always exercise with a partner trained to treat the condition.
5. Always wear a Medicalert bracelet or necklace.

❏❏ **What is the laboratory definition of exercise induced hematuria?**

Greater than three (3) red blood cells per high power field.

❏❏ **What are false positive causes of hematuria in athletes?**

1. High specific gravity rendering a positive test with less than 3 red blood cells per high power field.
2. Menses.
3. Hematospermia.

❏❏ **Exercise induced hematuria is most common in which two groups of athletes?**

Endurance runners and swimmers.

❏❏ **What is the first step in evaluating exercise induced hematuria in an otherwise asymptomatic athlete?**

Repeat the urinalysis in 24 - 48 hours after an exercise free time period.

❏❏ **What restrictions are placed on the athlete with exercise induced hematuria?**

No restrictions are necessary.

❏❏ **What percent of athletes demonstrate exercise induced proteinuria?**

70 - 100 % in studies.

❏❏ **What is the "normal" time course of exercise induced proteinuria?**

Proteinuria may occur within 30 minutes of exercise and resolves within 24 - 48 hours.

❏❏ **What is the range of exercise induced protein excretion?**

100 - 300 mg/ day (2 + to 3 + on dipstick).

❏❏ **What restrictions are placed on the athlete with exercise induced proteinuria?**

No restrictions are necessary.

❏❏ **What percent of healthy adolescents have mild proteinuria unrelated to exercise?**

10%.

❏❏ **What are the physiologic causes of benign, transient asymptomatic proteinuria?**

Increased glomerular permeability and decreased tubular resorption.

❏❏ **How can renal function be calculated from urine protein: creatinine ratio?**

24 hour urine protein ($gm/M^2/day$) = 0.63 x (Urine Protein/ Creatinine).
Normal = $\leq$ 1.0 gram.

❏❏ **In what percent of athletes has exercise induced hematuria been reported?**

11% - 100% The degree increases with intensity and duration of exercise.

❏❏ **How does microtrauma cause hematuria in athletes?**

Repetitive trauma to the genitourinary system due to high impact or high stress activities e.g. commonly seen with internal contusion of an empty bladder whereby the posterior strikes the fixed trigone.

❏❏ **What is "pseudohematuria"?**

Pseudohematuria is the absence of actual red blood cells. Common causes are:

1. Foods (beets & berries).
2. Artificial food coloring.
3. Hemoglobinuria.
4. Myoglobinuria.
5. Drugs (phenazopyridine, rifampin).

❏❏ **List pathological causes of true hematuria found in athletes.**

1. Urinary tract infection.
2. Urethral foreign body.
3. Post streptococcal glomerulonephritis.
4. Interstitial nephritis and papillary necrosis (NSAID's, creatine).
5. Alport's syndrome.
6. Sickle cell disease with sickling in the renal medulla.

7. Coagulopathies secondary to hepatotoxic substances.
8. Thrombocytopenia secondary to platelet abnormalities or disseminated intravascular coagulation.
9. Renal vein thrombosis secondary to blood doping or erythropoietin.

❑❑ How common are heartburn and gastroesophageal reflux?

They occur in 10 % of recreational runners and are more common in inexperienced athletes.

❑❑ How common is exercise induced gastrointestinal bleeding?

This occurs in 20% of endurance runners and the stomach is the most common site.

❑❑ What are causes of gastric bleeding with exercise?

1. Mechanical injury to the gastric fundus secondary to the shearing forces of the diaphragm and the gastrophrenic ligaments producing mucosal bleeding
2. Shunting of splanchnic blood flow and relative ischemia with mucosal bleeding

❑❑ Describe some non pharmacologic treatments for upper gastrointestinal symptoms in athletes.

1. Temporary decrease in high intensity exercise.
2. Anti reflux treatment regimen.
3. Reducing high fat meals prior to exercise.
4. Ingesting low osmolar, cool solutions during exercise.
5. Avoiding medications known to precipitate upper gastrointestinal symptoms, e.g. NSAID's.

❑❑ What are non pharmacologic treatments for the gastrointestinal symptoms?

1. Emphasis conditioning which decreases symptoms.
2. Train at different time of day (some have only morning symptoms).
3. Avoid eating 2-3 hours before exercise.
4. Limit caffeine containing foods and supplements.
5. Altering the timing of food ingestion to avoid gastrocolic reflex.
6. Limit fiber in diet.
7. Consider an elemental diet in some athletes.
8. Avoid sorbitol or mannitol.
9. Avoid large doses of Vitamin C.
10. Adequate hydration prior to exercise.
11. Maintaining adequate fluid ingestion prior to thirst stimulation to avoid the vicious cycle of dehydration diarrhea dehydration.
12. Utilizing appropriate fluids (5 - 8 % glucose will sodium facilitate absorption).
13. Consider temporarily reducing exercise intensity; then gradually resume.

❑❑ What percent of runners experience lower gastrointestinal symptoms with exercise?

30%.

❑❑ **What are possible causes of a decrease in transit time in the lower gastrointestinal tract in athletes?**

Direct effect of exercise.
Exercise in the upright position.
Dietary changes - increase in fiber and residue.
Adoption of performance enhancing diets - high dose minerals and Vitamin C.

❑❑ **T/F: The patient with a repaired atrial septal defect should have a normal exercise capacity.**

True.

❑❑ **T/F: During exercise patients with hypertrophic cardiomyopathy are at increased risk of sudden cardiac death.**

True.

❑❑ **T/F: Patients who have had a repair of their tetralogy of Fallot have an increased risk of sudden cardiac death.**

True.

❑❑ **T/F: The number one etiology of sudden cardiac death in adults with congenital cardiac disease is congenitally corrected transposition of the great vessels.**

True.

❑❑ **T/F: In a patient with congenital heart disease exercise will increase pulmonary artery pressure.**

True.

❑❑ **T/F: In a patient with repaired congenital heart disease myocardial dysfunction would be expected to worsen in response to exercise.**

True.

❑❑ **T/F: In a patient with congenital heart disease the cardiac output should be affected by the disease.**

True.

❑❑ **T/F: In a patient with a left to right shunt the oxygen consumption will increase in response to exercise.**

True.

❑❑ T/F: The presence of a large aorta to pulmonary artery collateral blood vessel would likely decrease the exercise capacity of the individual.

True.

❑❑ T/F: Patients with hypertension at rest and coarctation of the aorta should not be permitted to participate in competitive sports.

True.

❑❑ T/F: A history of syncope in a patient with hypertrophic cardiomyopathy is a contraindication to competitive sports.

True.

❑❑ T/F: Patients with borderline hypertension may participate in sports.

True.

❑❑ T/F: A patient with a congenital coronary artery fistula may show ischemic changes with exercise secondary to a coronary steal.

True.

❑❑ T/F: Patients with isolated pulmonary valve stenosis who have had prior pulmonary valvotomy should demonstrate normal exercise tolerance.

True.

❑❑ T/F: A hyperdynamic left ventricle is a common cause of post operative hypertension with exercise in patients with coarctation of the aorta.

True.

❑❑ T/F: A patient with severe aortic stenosis with a gradient of 45 mmHg should be prohibited from participating in a competitive sporting event.

True.

❑❑ T/F: The major source of energy for exercising muscle above the anaerobic threshold is anaerobic glycolysis.

True.

❑❑ T/F: The appearance of a malignant arrhythmia is an indication to terminate an exercise stress test in a patient with a repaired Tetralogy of Fallot.

True.

❏❏ **T/F: The hypoxic response in a patient with unrepaired congenital cyanotic heart disease is characteristically more severe with exercise as compared to the at rest response.**

True.

❏❏ **T/F: Patients with Tetralogy of Fallot without surgical correction demonstrate an increased ventilatory response to exercise.**

True.

❏❏ **T/F: Patients with Tetralogy of Fallot have reduced maximal exercise heart rates.**

True.

❏❏ **T/F: Following the Fontan procedure, aerobic capacity is increased from preoperative values.**

True.

❏❏ **T/F: Following the Fontan procedure, cardiac response to exercise is subnormal.**

True.

❏❏ **T/F: Systolic blood pressure that falls during progressive exercise demonstrates decreased cardiac output.**

True.

❏❏ **T/F: During exercise testing intracardiac shunts may reverse.**

True.

CLINICAL SPORTS MEDICINE

MUSCULOSKELETAL REHABILITATION

❑❑ **What nerve is involved in carpal tunnel syndrome?**

Median nerve.

❑❑ **In a patient with rotator cuff pathology, which shoulder movement is generally affected?**

Abduction.

❑❑ **Identify the syndrome most commonly associated by habitually carrying the shoulder lower than normal, so that the brachial plexus is subjected to abnormal stretch and pressure?**

Thoracic outlet syndrome.

❑❑ **What does physical therapy for patients with thoracic outlet syndrome involve?**

Toning and strengthening the elevators of the scapula so that the patient carries the shoulder higher.

❑❑ **What type of splint is recommended for an athlete with carpal tunnel syndrome?**

Cock up splint.

❑❑ **What term is used to describe damage to the lower part of the brachial plexus (C8, T1) as a result of grabbing a bar to break a fall?**

Klumpke's paralysis.

❑❑ **In Klumpke's paralysis, which part of the arm is affected?**

Distal portion (hand).

❑❑ **What are the two most common lesions in tissues joining the shoulder joint?**

RTC tears (especially the supraspinatus).
Rupture of the long head of the biceps.

❏❏ **What is the clinical consequence of paralysis of the serratus anterior muscle?**

Winging of the scapula.

❏❏ **Which nerve is damaged when an athlete is noted to have scapular winging?**

The long thoracic nerve.

❏❏ **Where do you expect to elicit pain and tenderness when examining a patient with "tennis elbow"?**

Lateral aspect of the elbow.

❏❏ **Which nerve is damaged in " wrist drop"?**

Radial nerve.

❏❏ **Why do infections within the tendon sheath of the little finger or that of the thumb present themselves at the wrist?**

Because of the continuity between the sheath finger tendons (1st, 5th) and the wrist.

❏❏ **What results would you expect from EMG and muscle enzyme studies in an athlete with steroid myopathy?**

Normal EMG and muscle enzymes.

❏❏ **What type of electrolyte abnormalities are associated with periodic paralysis (disorders characterized by recurrent attacks of flaccid weakness)?**

Abnormally high or low serum potassium concentrations.

❏❏ **A crush/ pressure injury to a muscle as well as vigorous exercise can result in a brown rust colored urine. What is this conditioned called?**

Myoglobinuria.

❏❏ **Fractures of the neck of the femur often tear which structure and make healing more difficult?**

Blood vessels.

❏❏ **What type of range of motion is normally found in the knee joint besides flexion and extension?**

Hyperextension.

❏❏ **Which movements are affected in a runner with injury to the tibial medial collateral ligament and anterior cruciate ligaments?**

The runner will be unable or limited in his attempt to change course suddenly.

❑❑ **How will severe weakness in the gluteal muscles affect the pelvis?**

Severe sagging of the pelvis on the opposite side resulting in gait difficulties.

❑❑ **In patients who elect not to have surgical repair of torn collateral or cruciate ligaments, the stability of the knee depends on which structures?**

Supporting muscles of the knee (quads/hamstring).

❑❑ **The common peroneal nerve is easily injured at its location near the fibular head. What is the resulting deficit?**

Foot drop.

❑❑ **What condition results from an imbalance among the muscles in the foot and can severely distort the foot?**

Club foot (Talipes).

❑❑ **Where does true hip pain generally localize?**

The groin.

❑❑ **Where does trochanteric bursitis generally localize?**

The lateral hip.

❑❑ **What does the finding of tenderness on palpation of the knee joint line suggest?**

Meniscal tear.

❑❑ **Which groups of muscles are involved in tennis elbow (pain and tenderness in the lateral epicondyle)?**

Forearm extensors and pronators.

❑❑ **Which muscle group is involved in golfer's elbow (pain and tenderness in the medial epicondyle)?**

Forearm flexors.

❑❑ **What is the most common peripheral neuropathy of the hand and wrist?**

Carpal Tunnel syndrome.

❑❑ **T/F: Complex regional pain syndrome I and II (reflex sympathetic dystrophy, shoulder hand syndrome) usually follows some type of noxious event such as CVA, fracture, nerve injury.**

True.

❏❏ **What is the most common cause of complex regional pain syndrome I and II?**

Trauma.

❏❏ **What anatomical structure is involved in Dupuytren's contracture?**

Thickening of palmar fascia.

❏❏ **What major musculoskeletal changes are seen with advancing age?**

Decreased muscle mass.
Increased body fat content.
Decreased total body water.

❏❏ **Identify signs of excessive exercise/therapy in patients with arthritic conditions?**

Post exercise pain of greater than two hours.
Undue fatigue.
Increased weakness.
Decreased range of motion.
Increased joint swelling.

❏❏ **What diagnosis is suggested in an athlete with multiple tender musculoskeletal points in the neck, back and extremities, along with fatigue, sleep disorder and decreased aerobic capacity?**

Fibromyalgia.

❏❏ **What does a normal rating in the manual muscle test signify?**

The muscle being tested is able to take full resistance.

❏❏ **What is the primary goal of physical rehabilitation?**

Restoration of function following physical impairment.

❏❏ **List some disadvantages of utilizing heat (hot packs) in musculoskeletal therapy?**

Increased swelling / Edema.
Accidental burns.

❏❏ **List some advantages of utilizing heat (hot packs) for musculoskeletal therapy.**

Increased tissue elasticity (decreased stiffness, increased relaxation and analgesia).

❏❏ **List some of the significant advantages of utilizing cold therapy for musculoskeletal rehabilitation.**

Increased analgesia.

Increased swelling.
Decreased spasm.
Decreased metabolic rate.
Decreased enzyme activity.

❏❏ **List significant disadvantage of cold therapy for musculoskeletal rehabilitation.**

Increased stiffness.
Decreased tissue elasticity.

❏❏ **In the arthritic joint, what type of force should be avoided across the arthritic joint?**

High restrictive forces.

❏❏ **How does aquatic therapy benefit athletes with pain syndromes?**

Decreased muscle activity and relaxation.
Decreased joint compression.

❏❏ **Name some adverse effects of forceful muscle stretching.**

Increased joint inflammation.
Tendon rupture.
Joint subluxation.
Fracture of osteoporotic bone.

❏❏ **List some of the adverse effects of prolonged rest.**

Decreased strength, bone mass and coordination.
Increased stiffness in the periarticular structures.

❏❏ **Which laboratory studies would you expect to be positive in myofascial pain syndrome?**

None.

❏❏ **Herniated intervertebral discs in the lumbosacral spine may produce tenderness on which structures?**

Spinous process.
Paraspinal muscles.
Intervertebral joints.

❏❏ **T/F: Increased anterior mobility of the knee may indicate instability of the anterior cruciate ligament.**

True.

❏❏ **T/F: Increased posterior mobility of the knee may indicate instability of the posterior cruciate ligament.**

True.

❏❏ **Which physiological changes occur with aerobic training?**

Increased myoglobin with O_2 affinity.
Increased aerobic muscle enzymes.
Increased size and number of mitochondria.

❏❏ **When can an athlete begin weight bearing following an ankle sprain?**

Whenever he/ she is able to bear weight.

❏❏ **Name some therapeutic options for the care of a patient with plantar fasciitis.**

Stretching & strengthening exercises.
Proper shoes with or without orthotics.
Ice and nonsteroidal antiinflammatory.
Iontophoresis.

SPECIAL CONSIDERATION

YOUNG ATHLETES

❑❑ **A 12-year-old otherwise healthy competitive runner presents with a burning sensation in chest and rapid breathing 6 minutes into running her race. What is the most likely diagnosis?**

The most likely diagnosis is exercise-induced bronchospasm (EIB). This condition often occurs at 6-10 minutes of intense exercise. Symptoms may vary from difficulty breathing with exercise, chest tightness, wheezing, coughing, or chest pain.

❑❑ **How does one diagnose exercise-induced bronchospasm (EIB)?**

An exercise provocation test is the diagnostic test of choice. Pulmonary function tests are performed at rest and once again after exercise. The subject exercises on a treadmill or cycle ergometer at 70-80% of predicted maximal heart rate. (The upright posture is most likely to induce a bronchoconstriction). The pulmonary function tests are then measured at 5, 10, and 15 minutes post exercise. EIB is defined as a drop of 15% or more of pulmonary function tests especially FEV1.

❑❑ **If the exercise provocation test is negative, and there is still a high suspicion of EIB what would you do?**

One can presumptively treat as EIB by premedicating with a bronchodilator. You can also perform the exercise provocation test under cold conditions. Sometimes exercise in a cold environment will trigger a bronchoconstriction. The young athlete may still test negative for EIB. There may be a combination of exercise and environmental pollutants that may produce a bronchoconstriction.

❑❑ **Are there any training techniques that one could do to avoid EIB?**

For each athlete there is a refractory period, a time in which the athlete is not vulnerable to bronchoconstriction and can exercise to full capacity. The duration of this refractory period will vary according to the individual. Appropriate warm-up techniques to make best use of this refractory period are indicated. There should be an avoidance of exercise on extreme cold conditions and when there is a great deal of environmental pollutants.

❑❑ **What percent of asthmatics suffer from EIB? Can one have EIB and not asthma?**

80-90% of asthmatics suffers from EIB. 10% of the general population who do not have asthma suffer from EIB.

☐☐ **A 12-year-old high level soccer player (plays in three leagues at the same time, middle school team, town team, and travel team) has been complaining of generalized muscle soreness, fatigue, and nonspecific joint pains. The coach has commented that he is not playing up to potential; in fact his performance has diminished. His parents have noticed that he has become increasingly belligerent and is no longer spending time with family and friends. What is the most likely diagnosis?**

This is called overtraining syndrome. There comes a point, where there is too much training and not enough time for the body to rest and recover. One of the first things that happen is a chronic injury or an injury that doesn't heal (chronic knee, shin, or heel pain). There usually is a decrease in performance. There are other nonspecific physiological and behavioral changes. One's peak muscle performance or aerobic fitness may be compromised; more likely, the athlete cannot reproduce the same peak torque or several submax tests.

☐☐ **Are there any blood tests that aid in the diagnosis of overtraining syndrome?**

Muscle enzymes—CPK, SGOT, or SGPT—may be markedly elevated. This is not diagnostic. One however, must rule out any systemic disease or cancer before labeling the young athlete as suffering from overtraining syndrome.

☐☐ **What is the treatment for overtraining syndrome?**

There are several treatment options for overtraining syndrome. A 50% reduction in training is recommended for a period of 2 to 12 weeks. A more extreme approach would be to take time off completely from the sport for 3 to 6 months. Both of these options would include a gradual increase in the training each week to get to the desired level.

☐☐ **How can physicians prevent young athletes from suffering from overtraining syndrome?**

The physician can help prevent overtraining syndrome by ensuring that the young athlete gains weight and grows in height, monitoring school performance, and screening for any significant mood changes. Communication with parent or coach is necessary to assure adequate improvement in performance in their sport. Those injuries that never seem to heal should be a hint that the athlete may be headed toward overtraining syndrome.

☐☐ **A 10-year-old female gymnast fell off the balance beam and hit herself awkwardly on the foot. She immediately complained of excruciating pain. She was seen by the orthopedist who diagnosed a possible 3rd/4th metatarsal fracture. She was casted and after several days began complaining of terrible pain. The cast was changed and she still complained of pain. Finally, she was placed on crutches and was unable to plantarflex or dorsiflex foot. What is the most likely diagnosis?**

The likely diagnosis is Reflex Sympathetic Dystrophy (RSD). This condition is characterized by severe pain and autonomic dysfunction. Children tend to have a very good prognosis whereas adults do not. The mechanism of the RSD may lead to severity of clinical symptoms. For example, the children usually suffer the RSD after a minor trauma. In contrast, adults often suffer the clinical entity after a compound fracture, surgery, burn, or electrical injury. There are numerous terms but a spectrum exists between mild pain and minor autonomic dysfunction to a totally dysfunctional extremity with edema, skin color changes, mottling, and a cold extremity. Two tip-offs as to the diagnosis are severe pain or worse pain with immobilization and undergoing months of physical therapy and still getting worse.

❑❑ Are there any diagnostic studies that are helpful in RSD?

Diagnostic studies are generally not helpful. X-rays in children are normal. MRI study may show nonspecific soft tissue swelling. Bone scans may be equivocal and show normal, increased, or decreased uptake.

❑❑ What is the treatment?

A treatment of intensive physical therapy employing desensitization techniques (deep tissue massage with cocoa butter, shaving cream, towel, wash cloth). Treatments with nortriptyline or Neurontin have proved to be beneficial. Sympathetic blocks are also helpful. If there is depression, anxiety disorder, or obsessive compulsive disorder then appropriate medication should be prescribed.

❑❑ A 12-year-old male soccer player has been complaining of pain in his heel for two weeks. He is limping toward the end of the game. Other than soccer his heel does not hurt him. What is the most likely diagnosis?

Sever's disease.

❑❑ What is the treatment for Sever's disease?

Treatment consists of decreasing the volume and intensity of impact activities. Heel cord stretching and ankle strengthening are also helpful. Heel cushions and over the counter orthotics may also be useful. Research is being done to examine the effects of the cleat on the incidence of heel pain in young soccer players.

❑❑ A 16-year-old cross-country runner has had difficulty breathing and has had to stop several races over the past several months at 6-7 minutes into a race. Parents and other teammates have noticed very noisy breathing. Treatment with bronchodilators has not been useful. What is the most likely diagnosis?

The most likely diagnosis is tracheomalacia. This condition most likely has been present since birth but has not presented itself until the athlete has reached this high level of exertion. Its symptom obviously mimic exercise induced bronchospasm. The keys to suspecting the diagnosis are unresponsiveness to bronchodilators and "noisy breathing".

❑❑ What is the treatment for symptomatic tracheomalacia with exercise?

Speech therapy emphasizing different breathing techniques.

❑❑ How does one make the diagnosis?

The diagnosis is difficult to make. A bronchoscopy during exercise may reveal the abnormality. A MRI of the airways may show abnormality in the trachea.

☐☐ **A 12-year-old boy, baseball pitcher, has had progressive worsening of medial elbow pain along with difficulty extending his elbow. He had similar symptoms one year ago. What is the diagnosis?**

The diagnosis is "Little League Elbow". The pathology here is medial epicondylar injury or medial apophyseal injury. If untreated and with continued throwing, this can lead to an avulsion fracture.

☐☐ **What is the treatment?**

Four to eight weeks of no throwing. During the time off from throwing, the young athlete should be involved with aerobic training at least two to three times per week and elbow/shoulder strengthening and flexibility.

☐☐ **What are some preventative measures?**

Counting pitch count, throwing 4-6 weeks prior to season, maintaining proper pitching technique, and biomechanics are all good preventative measures. A good strength and conditioning program 4-6 weeks prior to season is recommended. These consist of rotator cuff and scapular strengthening as well as shoulder and upper back flexibility exercises.

☐☐ **A 14-year-old has had progressive worsening shoulder pain and now hurts every time he throws. He can point specifically where the pain is. What is the likely diagnosis?**

The most likely diagnosis is Little League shoulder-proximal humeral epiphysitis. This is a stress fracture of the proximal humeral growth plate or Salter Harris I fracture.

☐☐ **How does Little League Shoulder differ from shoulder impingement or supraspinatus tendonitis?**

The location of the pain is quite different. Shoulder impingement occurs under the subacromial notch while Little League shoulder is lower down over the proximal humeral growth plate.

☐☐ **What is the treatment for Little League Shoulder?**

4-6 weeks of no throwing. Aerobic conditioning should be worked on, elbow/shoulder/wrist technique and proper biomechanics.

☐☐ **A 12-year-old boy with spina bifida comes to your office for advice regarding upcoming Special Olympics. Are there any special precautions? Are they trainable? Do you encourage them to participate?**

Children with neuromuscular disabilities should be encouraged to participate in physical activity. They may participate but with certain precautions. They are more subject to overuse injury and more likely to suffer from a heat injury.

❏❏ **What are the benefits of exercise for children with a neuromuscular disease?**

They may become stronger, more aerobic. Most of all, they benefit from enhanced self-esteem.

❏❏ **Are children with neuromuscular diseases trainable?**

Children with neuromuscular disabilities are trainable. They do not, however, have as much of an improvement in aerobic fitness and muscle strength as the able bodied population. They expend more energy per muscle movement than the able bodied population.

❏❏ **Are children more prone to heat injury than adults?**

Children are more prone to heat injury than adults. They have a higher surface area to volume. In addition, their thirst mechanisms are not as well developed as that of adults. When children say they are thirsty they are already dehydrated.

❏❏ **Do children need to take special precautions when exercising in the heat when compared to adults? What specific recommendations are there?**

Children need to drink 8 ounces beyond their thirst level before beginning sports participation. They need to drink 4-8 ounces every 15 minutes.

❏❏ **What content of drink should a child have? Is water okay?**

Children prefer flavored drinks. They particularly enjoy the grape flavor and will drink more of a preferred flavor.

❏❏ **What specific precautions do you need to take with children with cystic fibrosis who are exercising?**

Children with cystic fibrosis are prone to heat injury, they lost more salt and electrolytes in their sweat. They are also more likely to suffer from bronchoconstriction.

❏❏ **How do you define fibromyalgia in children? Is it different than it is in adults?**

The diagnosis of fibromyalgia is quite different in adults than in children. The patient must have chronic pain (11 out of 18 trigger points) and other nonspecific complaints (headaches, altered bowel habits, difficulty sleeping). American College of Rheumatology. Children often have less than 8 trigger points.

❏❏ **What is the treatment?**

Treatment is controversial. All patients need to live a regulated lifestyle, eating every 2-3 hours, getting adequate sleep, minimizing stressors. There may be a clinical response to nonsteroidal anti-inflammatory medication. With significant sleep disturbance and more severe pain, tricyclic antidepressants or Neurontin may be prescribed. The child should try to remain in school and maintain normal activities.

❑❑ What is the outcome?

Children tend to do well and with whatever treatment course usually are significantly improved within one year.

❑❑ What is hypermobility syndrome?

Hypermobility syndrome is defined as meeting three out of five criteria (thumb opposition, genu recurvatum, elbow hyperextension, hand/palm hyperextension). This is often synonymous with ligamentous laxity. This occurs in about 10% of teenagers especially girls. They often present to sports medicine specialists with recurrent ankle sprain or knee pain.

❑❑ How do we distinguish it from genetic syndromes?

There are no other associated systemic disease or organ abnormalities. In Marfan's syndrome there are skeletal, ophthalmologic, and cardiac problems. In Erhler Danlos syndrome there is defects in the collagen.

❑❑ Can they participate in all sports? How do we treat them?

They can participate in sports. They are more prone to joint pains, dislocations of patella, shoulder, and recurrent ankle sprains. Gedalia, Hypermobility Syndrome. They can participate in sports. They need to strengthen the body part that is being used in the sport. For example in running sports, they need to strengthen their ankle and knee. In swimming, they need to strengthen their rotator cuff and scapula muscles.

❑❑ Do overweight children need to take specific precautions when exercising? Are they more prone to certain injuries or conditions?

They are more likely to suffer from problems with the heat. Adipose cells carry less water than non-fatty cells. They are more likely to suffer from joint pains (knee, shin, ankle due to the extra weight they are carrying).

❑❑ What sports would you recommend for an overweight child?

One should recommend sports in which weight will serve as an advantage: hockey, football. Swimming especially at a young age. Overweight children are more buoyant.

❑❑ Are there any specific precautions to take with a child with inflammatory bowel disease who wants to exercise?

They are anemic. They may fatigue more easily. If they are experiencing explosive bloody diarrhea they shouldn't be participating in a contact sport.

❐❐ **Are there any guidelines for establishing when an elite young athlete is doing too much?**

There are a number of guidelines. Is the athlete improving his performance? Is he or she gaining weight and growing in height? Does he or she appear to be happy? Is there a personality change? Are there frequent infections? Are there injuries that do not heal right away? Are there repeated stress fractures?

❐❐ **In what sports are you most likely to see thoracic outlet syndrome.**

Thoracic outlet syndrome may show up in sports where there is abduction and external rotation—swimming, tennis, volleyball, baseball.

SPECIAL CONSIDERATION

FEMALE ATHLETES

☐☐ **When should primary amenorrhea be evaluated?**

Primary amenorrhea (delayed menarche) should be evaluated when there have been no menses nor secondary sex characteristics by the fifteenth year. Primary amenorrhea should also be evaluated if there are no menstrual cycles by the sixteenth year regardless of the presence of secondary sexual characteristics.

☐☐ **When can secondary amenorrhea be diagnosed?**

After menses have been established for at least 6 months, secondary amenorrhea is diagnosed when menses cease for three to six months.

☐☐ **What is the risk of amenorrhea in exercising women?**

In exercising women there is a risk of amenorrhea ranging from 1- 44 %.

☐☐ **During what times of life do most menstrual disorders occur?**

Most menstrual disorders occur near menarche and menopause when anovulatory cycles are more common.

☐☐ **What is the average age of menarche?**

The average age of menarche is 12.8 years.

☐☐ **What is the most common cause of amenorrhea in exercising women?**

Pregnancy.

☐☐ **What is Russell's sign?**

Callous formation of the backs of the hands due to self induced vomiting.

☐☐ **What is suggested by the triad of amenorrhea, galactorrhea and headaches?**

Prolactin secreting tumor.

☐☐ **In the above patient, what is your diagnosis if the MRI of the pituitary is normal, but the prolactin level is high?**

Idiopathic hyperprolactinemia.

❑❑ What does a positive progesterone challenge test tell you?

The progesterone challenge test determines if there is enough estrogen present to proliferate the endometrium and whether the outflow tract (uterus, vagina) is competent. Bleeding confirms adequate activity of the ovary, pituitary, hypothalamus. If the test is positive the patient is considered anovulatory.

❑❑ How is a progesterone challenge test done?

The test is done by administering 10 mg of medroxyprogesterone acetate orally for 5-10 days.

❑❑ What does a negative progesterone challenge test tell you?

If the patient does not bleed after a progesterone challenge test either the outflow tract is at fault or the endometrium has not been proliferated by estrogen.

❑❑ What do high levels of FSH and LH indicate in an amenorrheic patient?

The problem lies with the ovary, such as premature ovarian failure.

❑❑ Should all patients under age 30 years with premature ovarian failure undergo chromosomal analysis?

All women under the age of 30 years with the diagnosis of ovarian failure deserve a chromosome analysis even if they are normal in appearance. There are certain types of chromosomal abnormalities particularly mosaicism with a Y chromosome that carries a significant risk of malignancy.

❑❑ What do low levels of FSH and LH in an amenorrheic patient indicate?

Low levels of LH and FSH point to a prepubertal state or hypothalamic and pituitary dysfunction such as is seen in the female athlete triad and anorexia nervosa.

❑❑ Does exercise delay menarche?

Girls who begin intensive exercise prior to menarche have their first menses delayed an average of five months for every previous year of training compared to sedentary similarly psychologically stressed controls.

❑❑ Why does exercise delay menarche and affect menses?

The etiology is not fully understood but is felt to be due to an interplay between training and other variables including genetics and nutrition.

❑❑ Can an exercising woman have normal cycles yet be anovulatory?

Exercising women may have a shortened luteal phase of less than 7 days, low LH, FSH and estrogen levels and intermittent or absent ovulation. So while the women appeared to be menstruating regularly they were in fact not having normal cycles.

❑❑ What are the three components of the Female Athlete Triad?

The three components of the female athlete triad are disordered eating, amenorrhea and osteoporosis.

❑❑ Can the female athlete triad occur in non-elite athletes?

It occurs not only in elite athletes but in physically active girls and women. Societal and internal pressures for women and sometimes men to maintain unrealistically low weight for their sport encourage behaviors that lead to this disorder.

❑❑ Is it true that there is a belief among female athletes and to a lesser extent their coaches and other athletic staff that the cessation of menses in certain sports is a reflection of an appropriately intensive degree of training?

This is a common misconception in the sports community and in fact the opposite is true; the presence of female athlete triad is actually associated with declining performance as well as medical and psychological injury.

❑❑ What sports are more likely to see the Female Athlete Triad (FAT)?

FAT is seen in sports where slimness (diving, swimming and running) or physical beauty (gymnastics, dance, water ballet) may contribute to a better score.

❑❑ What is the cause of amenorrhea in FAT?

The amenorrhea in this syndrome is due to a decrease of the pulsatile hypothalamic Gn-RH release, which then leads to a decreased pituitary LH release and suppression of the ovarian estrogen production. It has been postulated that an imbalance between the stress of exercise and the body's energy availability in the form of body fat and caloric intake cause the hypothalamus to malfunction.

❑❑ What is the prevalence of disordered eating in athletes?

The prevalence is between 15 – 62%.

❑❑ What are the DMS IV criteria for anorexia nervosa?

Anorexia nervosa is an intense fear of gaining weight or becoming fat, even through under weight; disturbance in the way in which one's body weight or shape is experienced; undue influence of body weight or shape on self evaluation; or denial of the seriousness of the current low body weight and a weight less than 85% of that expected for height and age; and amenorrhea.

❑❑ What percentage of hospitalized anorexics die of complications?

15%.

❑❑ What are the complications associated with anorexia nervosa?

Complications include dental problems, electrolyte disorders, cardiomyopathy and death.

❑❑ **At what percent of ideal body weight do menses resume?**

The resumption of menses occurs at approximately 90% of ideal body weight.

❑❑ **What are the two types of bulimia?**

Purging and non purging.

❑❑ **What do the non purging bulimics use to loose weight?**

They exercise excessively.

❑❑ **What are the characteristics of bulimia?**

Bulimics do not have a distorted body image but their self image is unduly influenced by their body shape or weight. They have periods of lack of control over eating and for example in a two hour period they can eat an amount of food that is considerably larger than others would eat in similar circumstances (binging). They purge by vomiting, laxatives and /or diuretics. They symptoms must be ongoing for three months.

❑❑ **What bone pathology must an amenorrheic hypoestrogenic athlete be screened for?**

The amenorrheic, hypoestrogenic athlete is at risk for osteoporosis AND stress fractures. Workup will demonstrate lower bone mineral density than age matched controls due to decreased bony deposition and premature bone losses.

❑❑ **Who should coordinate the treatment of FAT?**

Treatment requires a coordinated approach with the athlete, parents, coaches, nutritionist, psychiatry and primary care or sports physician. Depending on the severity of the symptoms the care can be managed as an outpatient if the athlete's life is not in danger.

❑❑ **How should the osteopenia be treated or prevented in the hypoestrogenic athlete?**

The hypoestrogenic athlete should be supplemented with estrogen and calcium until her menses recur. Oral contraceptives should be used if she is sexually active because she may still ovulate even though she is amenorrheic and is at risk for pregnancy. Otherwise 0.625 mg of conjugated estrogens daily with 10 mg of medroxyprogesterone acetate 10 days of each month are used. Calcium in the form of calcium carbonate at 1500 mg/day and 400 -800 IU / day of Vitamin D are added. Follow bone density scans each year.

❑❑ **Can an amenorrheic athlete get pregnant?**

Yes, the patient can still ovulate.

❑❑ **Can oral contraceptive pills be used to manipulate the menstrual cycle around competition?**

Yes, although there is a risk of breakthrough bleeding.

❏❏ **Other than pregnancy, what is the most common cause of primary amenorrhea in girls?**

Constitutional delay.

❏❏ **How are constitutional delay and FAT similar?**

Both have low FSH, LH and serum estradiol levels and do not bleed after a progesterone challenge.

❏❏ **How are constitutional delay and FAT different?**

A family history of a mother or sister with delayed secondary sex characteristics and menarche hints at constitutional delay. Constitutional delay should have no evidence of disordered eating and a normal bone density scan. Diagnosis in the unclear case may require a several month trial of decreased activity such as during the off season for the patient's particular sport to be certain.

❏❏ **When is it necessary to perform a karyotype in women athletes with amenorrhea?**

A good rule of thumb is to perform a karyotype on all women less than 5 feet in height with primary amenorrhea and in primary amenorrhea or prolonged secondary amenorrhea in a woman less than 30 years of age.

❏❏ **How is anabolic steroid use detected in female athletes?**

The diagnosis is made by finding clinical signs of androgen excess and by checking for elevated serum androgen levels.

❏❏ **Are women more likely to be injured than men?**

No. With equal training there is no increase in injury.

❏❏ **Can girls and boys compete together?**

Yes, if similar weights and until puberty.

❏❏ **Does pregnancy affect athletic performance?**

Not in the first trimester. In fact there are reports of ergogenic benefits in early pregnancy but no control trials.

❏❏ **Does exercise improve bone density?**

No, it only maintains it.

❑❑ **What are the ACOG guidelines for exercise during pregnancy?**

Frequency : Regular (3/week) better than intermittent.
Position : Avoid supine position after first trimester, avoid prolonged standing.
Intensity: Stop when fatigued.
Type: Non weight bearing preferred, avoid possibility of loss of balance.
Avoid Valsalva.
Precautions: Adequate calories and fluids; watch for overheating.

❑❑ **How many extra calories per day are required during pregnancy?**

300 kcal/day.

❑❑ **What is the safe upper limit of normal heart rate for a pregnant patient?**

140 -160 bpm.

❑❑ **What are contraindications for exercise during pregnancy?**

Significant heart disease.
Cervical incompetence.
Uterine bleeding.
Ruptured membranes.
Intrauterine growth retardation.
Fetal distress.
One or more previous miscarriage.
Pregnancy induced hypertension.
Uncontrolled medical condition, i.e. diabetes.
Severe anemia.

❑❑ **What physiologic changes that occur during pregnancy affect exercise?**

Altered center of gravity, balance.
Ligamentous laxity.
Nerve compression from fluid retention.
Orthopedic problems due to all of the above.

❑❑ **Should hot tubs be avoided by pregnant athletes?**

A pregnant woman's body temperature should not exceed 100.4 especially after the first trimester.

SPECIAL CONSIDERATION

DISABLED ATHLETES

❏❏ **How many children in the United States have some kind of chronic condition?**

Current estimates are that 15 – 20 million children in the United States have some kind of chronic condition. Severe health conditions that are likely to require extensive daily care taking affect between one million and two million children.

❏❏ **What percent of children in the United States are thought to have some functional limitation due to chronic medical issues or disabilities?**

Approximately 5 – 10 % of children in the United States are thought to have some functional limitation due to chronic medical issues or disabilities.

❏❏ **How many Americans have an impairment that substantially affects major life functioning?**

Forty three million Americans have an impairment that substantially affects major life functioning.

❏❏ **How is the American Academy of Pediatrics' concept of the medical home applicable to children with disabilities?**

The American Academy of Pediatrics' concept of the Medical Home is directly applicable to children with disabilities. General medical care for all children needs to be accessible, family centered, continuous, comprehensive, coordinated, compassionate and culturally competent. It is in this framework that the health care provider can help children with disabilities and their families to become meaningfully involved in athletic activities.

❏❏ **What sports related issues should be discussed by the primary care physician?**

Comprehensive primary care should include the discussion of athletic participation and regular exercise.

❏❏ **Are sports activities important to the families of children with disabilities?**

Yes. The families of children with disabilities consistently report the importance of community based recreation programs.

❏❏ **Is consultation with other professionals often necessary for successful sports participation for people with disabilities?**

Yes. It is often necessary for the health care provider to communicate with other professionals, both medical and non medical, to ensure successful sports participation. Discussion and coordination with appropriate personnel including occupational, physical and speech therapists, vision specialists, physical education teachers, psychologists, neurologists, neurosurgeons, orthopedists, physiatrists and other professional is often necessary.

❏❏ **How does the Americans with Disabilities Act relate to sports participation?**

The Americans with Disabilities Act is a broad sweeping civil rights legislation that insures the rights of people with disabilities. The law encourages the full inclusion of children and adolescents with disabilities in activities with their peers without disabilities and calls for reasonable accommodations to help the child fully participate.

❏❏ **What are some of the complex medical issues present in children with disabilities?**

Children with disabilities have many complex medical problems. The following chart summarizes these problems:

Associated problems of Children with Disabilities

Cognitive delays	Hearing impairment
Communication deficits	Feeding difficulty
Learning problems	Emotional & behavioral problems
Seizure disorders	Orthopedic problems
Toileting difficulties	Other medical issues (cardiac, pulmonary, renal)
Visual difficulties	

❏❏ **What orthopedic issues need special consideration?**

Orthopedic issues such as scoliosis, hip subluxation or dislocation or "brittle bones" of osteogenesis imperfecta need special consideration.

❏❏ **What complicated psychosocial issues are common in the lives of children and adolescents with disabilities?**

Some children suffer with anxiety, depression and sadness. Self esteem issues are common and often impact on decision making. Different ways of dealing with the issues of independence and separation may interfere with athletic participation. Many children with disabilities live in relative social isolation and yet have almost no privacy in their personal lives because of their need for constant supervision. Peer relationships may suffer. School, family and social lives may be disrupted because of frequent hospitalizations. Behavioral and psychological problems are common and impact on athletic participation.

❑❑ **What are some of the psychosocial benefits of sports for children with disabilities?**

Psychosocial benefits are well known. Parents reports marked increases in self esteem. Increased socialization and opportunities for conflict resolution are very positive experiences. Sports allow children to feel good and proud about their accomplishments and to exhibit courage to themselves and others. Overall enjoyment and exposure to positive adult role models are also benefits. As with all children, it is also an outlet for physical energy and aggression.

❑❑ **What finding were reported in the Dykens and Cohen study concerning socialization and the Special Olympics?**

Their study found that social competence correlates with time spent in the Special Olympics regardless of age and IQ. Furthermore, Special Olympics athletes had more positive self perceptions.

❑❑ **What are the general reasons that regular physical exercise is particularly beneficial to the development of children with physical disabilities?**

The known benefits of cardiopulmonary fitness, decreased body fat, flexibility and increased muscle strength and endurance are critical to many children with disabilities. Increased mental alertness and psychological well being are additional benefits.

❑❑ **Why is increased fitness and exercise particularly important to people with disabilities?**

Individuals with disabilities need extra energy to use wheelchairs and orthotics. Awkward gait patterns are very tiring. Daily activities can be exhausting. Preventing obesity is important for people who use crutches to ambulate or who bear weight on weakened extremities. Preventing osteoporosis and strengthening bone structure and function is a critical aspect of exercise. Children with scoliosis and thoracic deformities may have compromised cardiopulmonary function and greatly benefit from fitness programs.

❑❑ **What about the psychological effects?**

Children who participate regularly in sports show less anxiety and depressive symptoms.

❑❑ **Summarize some of the obstacles and difficulties with athletic programs for children with disabilities.**

The following table summarizes these issues:

<u>Obstacles in Athletic Programming for Children with Disabilities</u>

Lack of disability specific opportunities	Inadequate transportation services
Overemphasis on winning	Poor toileting arrangements
Unrealistic parental expectations	Lack of appropriate medical evaluation
Liability issues	Lack of medical support
Lack of family support	Adolescent drop out
Inadequately trained coaches	Inadequate funding

❑❑ Why is it important to have disability specific opportunities for special athletes?

Many times, differing groups of athletes are combined into programs without regard to physical and /or mental characteristics. In a wheelchair basketball program, an individual with spastic quadraparetic cerebral palsy with upper and lower extremity involvement would be unable to compete fairly against someone with only lower extremity paralysis secondary to spinal cord injury.

❑❑ What is wrong with emphasis on winning and outcome rather than participation and social experience?

It will limit participation to the "best" and most competitive athletes. Many potential athletes will be discouraged from participating.

❑❑ Why are adolescents often unwilling to participate in athletic programs?

Some become self conscious of their disability and may lose their motivation to participate.

❑❑ In which disabilities are cardiac concerns of particular importance?

Cardiomyopathy and cardiac involvement secondary to pulmonary disease are common in primary neuromuscular disorders such as Duchenne's muscular dystrophy and spinal muscular atrophy. Cardiopulmonary evaluation is often necessary before sports participation.

❑❑ In which conditions is "too much exercise" contraindicated?

On occasion too much exercise may be contraindicated. This could be the case in certain children with severe pulmonary compromise secondary to scoliosis or severe anemia. Children with Duchenne's muscular dystrophy may have decreased strength and can easily overexercise. They may need repetitive, low intensity aerobic exercise.

❑❑ With which disabilities are environmental factors particularly important?

Environmental factors need to be considered especially in children who may have thermoregulatory difficulties as in familial dysautonomia, cystic fibrosis, severe dermatologic disorders and limb deficiencies.

❑❑ What are some examples of injuries that are more common in athletes with disabilities?

Disability specific injuries include fractures in children with osteogenesis imperfecta or osteoporosis. There may be overuse injuries such as tendonitis in children with tonal abnormalities such as cerebral palsy and dystonia.

❑❑ Which medical devices need special attention during athletic participation?

Extra care must be taken to avoid damage to ventriculoperitoneal shunts, central lines, gastrostomies, tracheostomies and respiratory equipment such as ventilators.

What is an adapted physical education program?

This is a specialized program for children who cannot participate in regular physical education. Adapted physical education programs are often included in special education programming as part of the individual education plan.

What are some of the sports options for children with disabilities?

Children may be "included" in scholastic intramural programs, interscholastic sports or community recreation leagues. The goals in "integrated" programs vary from intense competition to individual participation. Acting as a team manager may be extremely fulfilling for some adolescents. Many communities and organizations have "special" recreation leagues and programs.

What types of modifications are usually necessary for sports programs to be effective for children with disabilities?

These include cognitive, physical, behavioral and sensory considerations.

How can athletes with learning disabilities participate in sports activities?

Children with learning issues may have problems understanding rules, socializing and participating fully. Regular sports activities with extra support from coaches, teachers and counselors may suffice. Children with ADHD are often able to participate fully in programs with special modifications.

What is the Special Olympics?

Children with significant developmental delay (below average scores on intelligence tests) often need specially adapted programming. The Special Olympics (S.O.) is the most widely known and successful of these programs. The first S.O. games were held in 1968 under the auspices of Eunice Kennedy Shriver and the John P. Kennedy foundation. The goals are for children with developmental disabilities to have the opportunity to strengthen character, develop physical skills, display talents and fulfill human potential. Participants must be ≥ 8 years old. There is no fee. S.O. provides instruction, training and competition to developmentally disabled athletes. Activities are based on ability and include aquatics, track and field, gymnastics, bowling, skiing, volleyball, soccer, basketball, floor hockey, figure and speed skating, golf, cycling, tennis and roller skating. This program now consists on 1 million participants with 500,000 volunteers and 100,000 coaches in every state and many countries.

What are the principles of the Special Olympics?

The principles of the Special Olympics include activities that are appropriate for age and ability, the use of local volunteers, a family oriented approach and equality, respect and acceptance for all. Rules are adapted and the goal is to experience the joy of participation rather than winning.

❏❏ **What about children who are too disabled to participate in the Special Olympics?**

The Special Olympic (S.O.) motor activities training program (MATP) focuses on basic sensorimotor activities for those children whose level of functioning does not allow them to participate fully in S.O. The purpose of this program is to improve coordination and body control, increase exposure to sports and recreation, provide integration into community programs, improve sensory awareness and self concept and to prepare children for S.O.

❏❏ **What are some of the modifications necessary for physical disabilities?**

Modifications for physical disabilities include special skis and bicycles, adaptive bowling equipment, and wheelchair sports of all types. Adaptive winter sports such as skiing, snowboarding, skating and sledding are particularly popular. Wheelchair and adaptive sports include biking, bowling, floor hockey, fishing, hiking, races and events, golf, baseball and basketball. Wheelchair basketball can also be played with adapted baskets of varying heights and sizes. Special sleds and sticks are used in ice hockey. Aquatic sports such as swimming, water skiing and boating with special flotation devices and other adaptive equipment are especially popular because there is no undue pressure on joints and bones.

❏❏ **What are some modifications for sensory impairment?**

Programs of this type often stress multisensory experiences. Special adaptations include the use of a "beeper ball", brightly colored equipment, sign language, easily read signs and other visual prompts. Goalball, using a ball with four bells inside, is a unique sport for the visually impaired that has developed into an internationally popular event now being enjoyed by nondisabled individuals as well.

❏❏ **What are some additional popular sports opportunities for children with disabilities?**

Challenger Little League Baseball, Soccer, Horseback riding, dance, tennis, table tennis and karate.

❏❏ **Give an example of a model program for people with disabilities.**

The Empire Games for the Physically Challenged is an innovative model program in New York State that has been extremely successful. Participants are children 5-21 years of age. There are both competitive and noncompetitive sporting events. The classifications for participants are amputee, blind and visually impaired, cerebral palsy, deaf and hearing impaired, Les Autres (osteogenesis imperfecta, muscular dystrophy, arthrogryposis, dwarfism, and cardiac and pulmonary disorders) and spinal cord injury. Extensive care is taken for the competition to be fair.

❏❏ **What are some guidelines for counseling children and adolescents with disabilities about sports participation?**

The first consideration is the appropriateness of the suggested activity and its availability. The activity need to be proper for the child's age and developmental level and functionally useful. Furthermore, the child should be involved in the decision making process. The practical aspects of participation such as transportation and finances must be considered. Cognitive ability, social and behavioral skills and physical and sensory limitations must all be considered. Practical aspects of participation include the need for adaptive equipment and modifications. Risks need to be discussed openly and candidly and recommendations for appropriate equipment (glasses, helmets) should be made. The American Academy of Pediatrics has general guidelines on counseling children and adolescents about sports participation.

☐☐ Briefly describe the preparticipation exam for disabled athletes.

History includes cardiac symptoms, injuries, previous surgery, seizures and past participation experiences. Any medications should be reported and effects evaluated. A complete physical exam is necessary including blood pressure and a careful cardiac evaluation. Particular attention should be paid to the neurological and orthopedic exam and any limitations. Vision and hearing should be evaluated. Special problems such as single testicle or kidney, VP shunt or gastrostomy need to be addressed.

☐☐ What are some of the common characteristics of cerebral palsy that impact on athletic participation?

Tonal abnormalities (spasticity, athetosis and ataxia) are primary characteristics of cerebral palsy as are persistent primitive reflexes. Contractures are common. Cognitive, communication and perceptual deficits are frequent. Many individuals have seizures and may require specialized medications. Sensory and visual perceptual impairments are also common.

☐☐ How do these characteristics of cerebral palsy affect sports participation?

A large number of individuals with cerebral palsy participate in sports activities and need special considerations. Decreased exercise tolerance and possible lack of flexibility secondary to the tonal problems of spasticity, athetosis and ataxia need to be addressed. The effect of exercise on spasticity and problems of overuse must be considered. A well planned program including flexibility training and strength training can be successful. Contractures can limit range of motion and strength. Persistent primitive reflexes, (especially startle and asymmetric tonic neck) can interfere with performance. Consultation with a physical therapist or physiatrist may be necessary. Modifications are often made because of cognitive, communication and perceptual deficits. Seizure, while common in cerebral palsy is not usually a problem in athletic participation. Some medications used to treat spasticity may cause weakness and fatigue. Anticholinergic medication (for saliva control) may lead to overheating and excessive sweating.

☐☐ What is atlantoaxial instability (AAI) and how is it managed?

The most controversial aspect of sports participation for children with Down's syndrome is atlantoaxial instability. It is an especially common situation, as 15 % of children with Down's syndrome are affected. AAI is defined as increased mobility at the articulation of the first and second cervical vertebrae. Fortunately, symptomatic AAI is uncommon. The neurologic exam is diagnostic, as cervical x rays are of limited predictive value. Neurologic findings of significance include easy fatigability, abnormal gait, difficulty walking, neck pain, limited neck mobility, torticollis, incoordination, clumsiness, increased reflexes, clonus, positive Babinski, sensory changes and weakness. It is clear that a careful neurological exam or referral to a neurologist and / or neurosurgeon may be necessary for complete evaluation. The American Academy of Orthopedic Surgeons suggests that there be an initial screening X ray for diagnostic purposes and followup is needed. The Special Olympics still requires cervical X rays before participation. Most recent recommendation suggest avoiding activities like tumbling, diving, gymnastics, football and soccer in the presence of AAI.

What are some additional concerns of athletes with Down's syndrome?

Athletes with Down's syndrome need complete preparticipation evaluations as described above. Particular attention needs to be paid to ligamentous laxity and hypotonia. In particular pes planus and other foot problems are common. Foot orthotics may be necessary. Congenital heart disease and obesity are other problems that may need special attention.

What are some of the characteristics of athletes with spina bifida?

Individuals with spina bifida having varying degrees of spinal cord involvement and hydrocephalus. A ventriculoperitoneal shunt is common. Arnold Chiari malformation involving the upper spinal cord and base of the skull presents special challenges. There is paralysis of the lower extremities and sensory loss depending on the level of involvement. There is usually significant bowel and bladder dysfunction. Cognitive and learning problems as well as sensory and visual perceptual impairments are common. Medication is often taken for bladder control.

How are the concerns of athletes with spina bifida met?

Children with spina bifida raise special concerns when participating in sports activities. Excessive concerns over spinal cord involvement, which is central to the disability, are usually unnecessary. Children with spina bifida generally tolerate sports well. Any considerations of spinal cord involvement, such as tethering, should be coordinated with a neurologist or neurosurgeon. While damage to the ventriculoperitoneal shunt is possible, it is uncommon. Regular athletic helmet recommendations should be followed. Arnold Chiari malformation is of concern, much like atlantoaxial instability. Cervical spine precautions should be followed and similar sports avoided if it is present. Cognitive and learning problems, common in athletes with spina bifida may require adaptations to the rules. The musculoskeletal characteristics of spina bifida may be a problem. Osteoporosis and lack of sensation make the legs especially vulnerable to injury. Modifications for the wheelchair and orthotics need to be considered. While bowel and bladder dysfunction may be a nuisance during athletics, they are usually not major problems. They do however, dictate the need for accessible and appropriate toileting facilities. Anticholinergic medications used for bladder control can lead to overheating. Modifications for sensory and visual perceptual impairments may be necessary.

What are the concerns for children with Duchenne's muscular dystrophy and other myopathies?

Duchenne muscular dystrophy (DMD) is a rare disorder. Athletic participation should be encouraged throughout the life of children with DMD. Common factors affecting athletics are the underlying muscle weakness, obesity, respiratory compromise and the possibility of overwork weakness. The goals of athletic participation with DMD need to be modified somewhat. Maintenance of strength becomes a primary goal. It is difficult and often impractical to build up strength in children with progressive neuromuscular disorders. Because of the X linked recessive inheritance pattern of DMD, there are often overwhelming family issues which impact on the child's participation. These include the presence of another male family member, feelings of guilt and/ or depression and other psychosocial issues. Significant contractures and profound proximal weakness often require extensive athletic modifications. Scoliosis and restrictive pulmonary disease may impact on endurance as well. Cardiopulmonary consultation is often needed for extensive sports participation because of the possibility of cardiomyopathy from primary cardiac disease and chronic pulmonary disease.

❐❐ **How does the concept of overwork weakness relate to children and adolescents with Duchenne muscular dystrophy?**

Children with DMD should not exercise to the point of exhaustion due to the risk of muscle damage. The warning signs of overwork weakness, include feeling weaker rather than stronger within 30 minutes post exercise or excessive muscle soreness 24 – 48 hours following exercise. Other warning signs include severe muscle cramping, heaviness in the extremities and prolonged shortness of breath. Low impact aerobic exercise like walking, swimming and stationary bicycling seem to be effective and will improve cardiovascular performance and increase muscle efficiency and ultimately help fight fatigue. It is also beneficial in fighting depression, maintaining ideal body weight and improving pain tolerance. Consultation with therapists is often necessary in the presence of progressive muscle weakness.

SPECIAL CONSIDERATION

SENIOR ATHLETES

❑❑ **What percentage of the population is currently over 65 years?**

14%.

❑❑ **Which geriatric age category is proportionately growing the fastest?**

85 years and older.

❑❑ **What percentage of this population exercises regularly?**

About 30%, 58% are sedentary.

❑❑ **What happens to the temporal organization of physiologic rhythms with aging?**

Loss of spectral reserve, complexity, variability or 'bushiness' in heart rate, blood pressure, pulsatile secretions of hormones, EEG and auditory frequencies, postural sway and physiologic tremor. Homeostasis is replaced by homeostenosis.

❑❑ **With respect to the elderly what is the most reliable parameter for classification?**

Functional or physical capacity is much more reliable than chronological age.

❑❑ **What is one of the most reliable clinical signs of muscle strength and power?**

Gower's sign - the need to walk up one's thighs when asked to rise from a sitting position.

❑❑ **What happens to the maximal oxygen uptake as a person grows older?**

From the age of approximately 20 years onward there is a gradual decline in uptake averaging about 1 ml/kg-min per year (0.9% per year) which accelerates after 80 years. The rate of decline is significantly slower in trained athletes compared to sedentary populations. At all ages male oxygen uptake is higher than females.

❑❑ **How do athletes in endurance disciplines compare to nonathletes?**

At any age athletes have significantly higher maximal aerobic power than is found in the general population. An aerobically fit 70-year-old can outperform a sedentary 30-year-old.

❑❑ **What happens to heart rate with age?**

There is a gradual decline in maximal heart rate (10 bpm/decade).

❑❑ **What is the maximum heart rate for an 84 year old?**

Maximum heart rate (MHR)= 220-age+/- 12bpm. Therefore the MHR would be 136+/- 15bpm.

❑❑ **What impact does endurance training have on the heart?**

At any age regular endurance training produces a significantly greater left ventricular mass and volume. Heart size is larger in trained master athletes compared to sedentary counterparts.

❑❑ **What other changes occur with aging in the cardiovascular system?**

The stroke volume, passive filling, left ventricular diastolic reserve and peripheral oxygen extraction decreases, arterio-venous difference remains the same, and maximum cardiac output declines (6-8%/decade). The resting cardiac output and ejection fraction remain the same, and there is an increased dependence on atrial contraction.

❑❑ **What happens to blood pressure with aging?**

Systolic, diastolic and mean arterial pressures increase; however, diastolic pressure rises until sometime between 35-65 years and thereafter plateaus or declines. The etiology is increased stiffness of the arterial tree.

❑❑ **What is the most appropriate way to assess to aerobic power in the elderly?**

Measurement of the maximum oxygen uptake.

❑❑ **How is anaerobic power and capacity determined?**

An accurate measurement is not available. Lactate levels are an indirect measurement. Lactate levels are lower in trained individuals, and peak concentrations are lower in the elderly at any given percentage of maximal aerobic power. The anaerobic or lactate threshold occurs at a work rate, which represents 40-60% of the maximal oxygen uptake. The VO_2max is a better predictor of performance than the lactate threshold.

❑❑ **What impact does endurance training have on the pulmonary system?**

It reduces (normalizes) pulmonary ventilation at a given relatively high oxygen uptake.

❑❑ **Identify the changes that occur in the pulmonary system with aging.**

Total lung volume, vital capacity (25ml/yr), maximum voluntary ventilation, diffusing capacity, alveolar ventilation, PaO_2 (4mmHg/decade) and inspiratory (26 ml/yr) and expiratory (32 ml/yr) flow rates fall, residual and closing volumes (30-50% by age 70) increase. Elastic recoil is lost, respiratory muscle strength and surface area declines and compliance increases causing an increased feeling of breathlessness. Pulmonary blood flow is redistributed due to increased resistance and loss of small vessels. There is ventilation-perfusion mismatching.

❑❑ What changes occur in muscular strength with aging?

There is a significant reduction in dynamic and static strength after the age of approximately 50 years. The strength of a 65 year old person is, on average, 75-80% of that attained between the ages of 20 and 30, with a further decline to about 60% in back and leg muscles, and to 70% in arm muscles from 30 to 80 years of age. Strength rapidly drops off after 80 years of age. Power (strength/time) also declines by 0.6%/yr. Strength in the lower extremities is lost at a relatively faster rate than upper extremity strength.

❑❑ Relate muscle strength and mass with aging.

The decline in strength (10-15%/decade after 60 years) with age parallels the reduction in muscle mass (24-36% after 65 years of age).

❑❑ Are any muscles relatively spared from the effects of aging?

The diaphragm.

❑❑ What is the cause for reduced muscle mass?

Loss of muscle fiber number, perhaps down to 60% of the initial fibers, and a 50% decline in the size (cross-sectional area) of fast-twitch fibers (type II) by the eighth decade. Type I fibers (slow twitch) remain unchanged in number and size until after the seventh decade.

❑❑ What changes occur to the motor neuron unit?

There is a significant loss of motoneurons (1-3%/year after 60).

❑❑ What effect does training have on strength?

There is a gradual increase in the area of type II fibers followed by an increase in strength and power. There is a specificity in the training.

❑❑ Review the effect of weight training on the aged muscle.

Progressive resistance exercises is well tolerated by both robust and frail elderly persons and produces increases in tensile strength primarily especially eccentric (muscle lengthening) ones. Short term resistance training has modest or no effect on muscle mass. Improvements are not correlated with increases in muscle cross-sectional area.

❑❑ What changes occur to flexibility with aging?

There is a significant decline in flexibility with aging due to inactivity (muscle and tendon tightness) and degenerative disease.

☐☐ **What changes occur to body composition with aging?**

Muscle and bone mass decline and adipose tissue increases in both sexes until 65-70 years in males when adipose tissue declines.

☐☐ **What important endocrinologic changes occur with aging?**

Increased serum glucose (1%/decade after 20 years), increased plasma insulin (impaired insulin sensitivity, decreased growth hormone, testosterone and estrogen levels, glucose tolerance.

☐☐ **What important nervous system changes occur with aging that affect functional status?**

There is a decline in balance and proprioception resulting in a 30-40% increase in falls. There is a 1-15% decline in nerve conduction and a 37% loss in the number of spinal cord axons. Clinically, quickness is lost before flexibility and strength.

☐☐ **What effect does regular aerobic training have on lipid metabolism?**

Raises the absolute HDL level and the HDL/LDL ratio.

☐☐ **What effects does age have on trainability?**

Minimal, given sufficient frequency per week and intensity per session and training lasting about 20 weeks.

☐☐ **What are the general effects of regular exercise in the elderly?**

Improved quality of life as noted by increased strength, flexibility, bone mass, station, gait, coordination, and aerobic power and decreased blood pressure and low back pain. Psychosocially, there is improved sleep patterns, weight control, body image, social contacts, sense of independence and decreased depression and numbers of accidents. If regular aerobic training is begun in younger adulthood the incidence of coronary heart disease is reduced and longevity increased due to all-cause and cardiovascular mortality rate declines.

☐☐ **What is the major risk factor for sudden death in the elderly who exercise?**

Coronary artery disease which is often occult.

☐☐ **What is the recommended approach for clearing a healthy elderly patient?**

Performing an appropriate history (comorbid states, medications, smoking, alcohol use, prior injuries/rehab, occupation/hobbies) and focused clinical exam (musculoskeletal, cardiopulmonary) and resting 12 lead EKG.

☐☐ **When is it appropriate to perform a graded exercise test?**

The presence of 2 or more risk factors (hypertension, smoking, positive family history, impaired glucose tolerance, obesity or increased serum lipids), abnormal evaluation (signs/symptoms of cardiovascular disease) or EKG in a patient desirous of starting a moderate exercise program(40-60% functional capacity) or all elderly patients wanting to start a vigorous program (>60% VO_2max).

❑❑ How do the elderly handle heat stress?

Old age is associated with heat intolerance due to blunted thirst, impaired skin vasodilation, decreased sweat production with a greater threshold to initiate sweating and reductions in aerobic power and/or lack of acclimation. There is no conclusive evidence that advanced age per se is casually related to a dysfunction of the temperature regulatory system.

❑❑ Are the elderly at risk for hypothermia?

Yes, due to decreased muscle activity, glucose-induced thermogenesis, impaired vasoconstrictor response, less efficient shivering, and difficulty in discriminating temperature differences especially a delayed perception of being cold.

❑❑ Name the characteristics of heat stroke in the elderly.

Classical heat stroke is noted by its high temperature, the presence of comorbid states, anhydrosis, respiratory alkalosis, mild enzyme elevation and hyperuricemia and rarely rhabdomyolysis, disseminated intravascular coagulation and acute renal failure.

❑❑ What are the effects of high altitude on the aged?

Approximately 5% of high altitude trekkers are > 65 years. The elderly have a lower incidence and severity of acute mountain sickness and high altitude pulmonary edema when compared to the younger adults.

❑❑ What drug therapy is most appropriate for pain from degenerative joint disease?

Acetaminophen up to a 4gm maximum/day.

❑❑ What is the rate of bone loss after 55 years?

3-5% / year with trabecular losses greater than cortical. By 70 years of age females have lost 30-35% of their cortical bone and 50% of their trabecular mass with males losing 20% and 33% respectively.

❑❑ What factors are related to cortical bone thickness in elderly females?

Physical activity and previous use of estrogen. Regular exercise causes enhanced mineralization of the stressed bones in the aged.

❑❑ What is the impact of bedrest on musculoskeletal system?

1% / week decrease in vertebral mineral density and for every 2 days of bedrest one day of strength and aerobic training will be needed for return to baseline.

❏❏ **When does a bone scan become abnormal following a fracture?**

Within 12 hours.

❏❏ **What is the best technique to evaluate bone loss in the elderly?**

Dual photon absorptiometry (DEXA) is the method of choice for trabecular bone examination, since it is inexpensive, radiation dose is low and the vertebrae can be measured.

❏❏ **Name some important guidelines to avoid unnecessary injury.**

1. Keep resistance <80% of the 1 repetition maximum.
2. Exercise within the aerobic limits established by the exercise test.
3. Avoid weight lifting, running and jumping rope in selected patients.
4. Establish the target heart rate of 60-75% of the maximum heart rate.
5. Avoid isometrics in patients with CHF, CAD or hypertension.
6. Advise patients with visual or hearing impairments about the dangers of exercising without special precautions (e.g. traffic).

❏❏ **Does running, walking, or jogging cause degenerative joint disease?**

No.

❏❏ **Identify the components of an exercise prescription for the mature athlete.**

30 minutes or more of moderate intensity (3 to 6 METs) of physical activity on most, and preferably all days of the week. The program should be started slowly and progressed gradually in sedentary individuals.

❏❏ **What is the most important factor in the prescription?**

Intensity.

❏❏ **How is intensity determined?**

Intensity depends on the initial fitness level of the patient. It is difficult to determine since it is expressed as a percentage of the maximum heart rate, heart rate reserve or functional capacity. Two methods are used. One utilizes 60-90% of the MHR, which corresponds to 50-85% of the functional capacity. The second is the Karvonen method, which is preferred since variability in the athlete's resting heart rate is taken into account.

❏❏ **Utilizing the Karvonen formula, determine the training heart rate (THR) in an 86 year old with a pulse of 65 who desires a moderate exercise program.**

THR=[0.60 to 0.90 x (MHR - RHR)] + RHR where MHR=maximum heart rate, THR=training heart rate and RHR=resting heart rate and 0.60 to 0.90 represents the level of intensity. So, for our patient the THR= 0.75 x (134 – 65) + 65=117bpm.

What options are available for patients with disabilities?

METS (metabolic equivalent units) can be used. 1 MET= 3.5 ml/kg/min oxygen consumed at rest in a sitting position. Maximum MET= VO2max/3.5. Low intensity training should utilize 0.5 MMET whereas high intensity programs should incorporate 0.85 MMET. Any number of tables should be consulted for the MET cost of various activities.

What is the ideal duration of exercise?

20-60 minutes of continuous aerobic activity at a moderate intensity. A 5-10 minutes warm-up and cool-down period should also be included.

Describe the frequency of exercise bouts.

A minimum of 3 sessions/week is necessary to achieve an aerobic effect for the average adult. Obese and functionally impaired adults (<3 METs) should be prescribed multiple 5-10 minute sessions several times/day until they are able to endure longer sessions. Exercise sessions should not exceed 5 days/week and not more than 2 sessions/week should be intense.

T/F: Exercising 7 days a week incrementally improves aerobic power?

False. And such a schedule is likely to lead to overuse injuries. The one exception is the obese adult who requires multiple low-intensity sessions to reduce body fat.

What is the appropriate aerobic exercise mode?

Activities that use large muscle groups in a continuous rhythmic manner (e.g. cycling, skating, cross-country skiing, swimming, rowing, walking/jogging/running) are appropriate for aerobic conditioning.

What is recommended for strength training?

The major muscle groups (e.g. legs/thighs, arms/forearms, shoulders, chest and back) should be exercised 2-3 times/week for improvement and once/week for maintenance. 8 (60% max 1 rep) repetitions in 3 to 4 sets for each muscle group is traditionally recommended although newer evidence suggests that fewer repetitions and sets utilizing less weight and done on a 10-20 count produces similar results. Levels of intensity >80% of the 1 rep max have no benefit and only risk for cardiovascular and musculoskeletal injury. Substantial gains in strength commonly occur within 8-12 weeks and plateau thereafter.

Identify those conditions requiring moderation of activity.

Significant musculoskeletal injuries.
Extreme cold, especially associated with significant wind-chill.
Extreme heat and high relative humidity.
Following heavy meals.
Altitudes >6000 feet.

❑❑ **Name the important conditions requiring supervised exercise training and testing**

Recent myocardial infarction or post-CABG.
Use of a pacemaker (fixed or demand).
Severe hypertension.
Intermittent claudication.
Use of inotropic or chronotropic medications.
Occurrence of ST segment depression at rest.
Presence of morbid obesity with multiple coronary risk factors.

❑❑ **Identify those conditions requiring activity moderation/prescription caution.**

Exercise-induced cold.
Chest pain.
Infection.
Prolonged, unaccustomed physical activity.
Irregular heart rate.
Conduction disturbance (LBBB, 3rd degree AV block, bifascicular block with or without first degree block).

❑❑ **How should the mature athlete monitor the program?**

Measurement of the radial pulse for 6 seconds immediately after stopping exercise which has been ongoing for 10 minutes and multiplying by 10 (or adding a zero).

❑❑ **Discuss the parameters for exercise program progression.**

The rate of progression depends on the athlete's age, physical capacity, exercise goals and overall health status. Only one variable should be modified in any one session. The initial phase (50-60% VO$_2$max gradually increasing 2-3 minutes every 1-2 weeks up to 20 minutes/session) lasts an average of 6 weeks (2-10 week range). The improvement phase (70-85% VO$_2$max incrementally increasing 2-5 minutes up to 30-45 minutes/session 3 to 5 times/week) can be up to 6 months or more and the maintenance phase (70-85% VO$_2$max for 30-45 minutes 3 to 5 times/week) for the following 6 months.

❑❑ **What is the basis for progression?**

Subjectively there should be a decrease in fatigue and perceived exertion; improved movement patterns and more relaxed body language. Objectively, there should be a decrease in the RHR (3-8bpm) at a given intensity; voluntary adaptation of a faster pace and improved functional capacity.

❑❑ **What are the most common injuries in the mature athlete?**

In rank order they are: tendonitis, patellofemoral pain syndrome, osteoarthritis, strain and sprain.

❑❑ **Where do most injuries occur?**

In rank order they are: knee foot, leg, shoulder and ankle.

❑❑ **Why do injuries most commonly occur?**

Rapid progression of an exercise program.

❑❑ **Identify the components of a healthy diet for a mature athlete.**

Calories: 1400kcal/day for females and 1700kcal/day for males 60-70% of the diet made of carbohydrates, <30% fat, and 0.8-1.5gms/kg/day protein (110-20%) depending on the intensity of the program.

❑❑ **What is the current recommendation for sedentary older persons?**

Increased physical activity (180 minutes/week) and not to perform strenuous exercise. Jogging/running is not recommended for persons who have not run in many years.

❑❑ **How often should flexibility training occur?**

Daily.

❑❑ **Can balance be improved?**

Yes. Balance is plastic and is improved through Tai Chi training. A reduction in fall rates has been noted.

SPECIAL CONSIDERATION

INFECTIOUS CONCERNS

❏❏ T/F: An examining physician may disqualify a wrestler from competition if he/she believes there is presence of a communicable disease that makes participation inadvisable.

True.

❏❏ T/F: Daily disinfection of wrestling mats and equipment has been demonstrated to decrease rates of bacterial skin infection.

True.

❏❏ A student returns from wrestling camp with cluster of painful vesicular lesions on his left shoulder. What is the most likely diagnosis?

Herpes gladiatorum; a local inoculation of Herpes simplex virus obtained through close contact.

❏❏ T/F: Wrestlers with local herpetic skin infections may safely return to competition when the lesions become dry and crusted, even if they have not totally resolved.

True.

❏❏ T/F: A basketball player is diagnosed with meningococcal meningitis one day after the team traveled by bus to a game. All of his teammates and the coaching staff should immediately receive meningococcal vaccine.

False.

❏❏ T/F: A football player is diagnosed with pneumococcal meningitis. No prophylactic therapy is indicated for his teammates and coaches.

True.

❏❏ T/F: Close contacts of an athlete diagnosed with meningococcemia may be effectively prophylaxed with rifampin, ceftriaxone or ciprofloxacin if they are >18 years of age.

True.

❑❑ **T/F: A football player is found to have a positive PPD (>15 mm induration) on screening physical examination. A chest x-ray is negative. The athlete should be excluded from the team until he has completed 4 weeks of isoniazid (INH) therapy.**

False.

❑❑ **A football player complains of acute right upper quadrant pain after a tackle. His vital signs are stable and an abdominal ultrasound reveals a small hematoma of the spleen within the capsule. A CBC reveals a hematocrit of 41% and white blood cell count of 13,000 /mm^3 with 17% atypical lymphocytes. What is the most likely diagnosis?**

Infectious mononucleosis. Although typically mononucleosis presents with pharyngitis, lymphadenitis, fatigue and fever in association with splenomegaly, splenic rupture may be the initial presentation of the infection.

❑❑ **T/F: The child in the above question requires emergency splenectomy.**

False. If stable, the patient may be monitored at bed rest and possibly avoid splenectomy.

❑❑ **T/F: An athlete diagnosed with acute infectious mononucleosis may return to participation in contact sports in 1 to 2 months after the onset of symptoms and when his (her) splenomegaly has resolved.**

True.

❑❑ **A 16-year-old athlete from Central America, in the United States for 3 years, suffers a deep laceration on his leg after falling in the dirt. His tetanus status is unknown. After cleaning the wound, proper prophylaxis against tetanus would include.**

Administration of tetanus immune globulin [T.I.G.] and tetanus toxoid.

❑❑ **T/F: In the above setting, if his medical record documents at least three prior doses of tetanus toxoid with the last dose given 7 years ago, no additional tetanus preventive therapy is indicated.**

False. Although T.I.G. is not indicated, in the face of a dirty wound an additional dose of tetanus toxoid should be administered if it is >5 years since the last dose.

❑❑ **T/F: An athletic team's bus driver is diagnosed with cavitary tuberculosis. Proper management of team members would include prophylactic isoniazid (INH) for 3 months pending results of tuberculin skin tests place at time of exposure and follow up at 3 months.**

False.

❑❑ **T/F: A student who is Hepatitis B surface antigen positive should not be allowed to participate in contact sports.**

False.

❏❏ **A basketball player suffers a bite injury with deep puncture marks to the knuckles of his hand. What would be appropriate oral antibiotic therapy to prevent infection in this situation?**

Amoxicillin-clavulanate [Augmentin].

❏❏ **In the scenario above if the patient were penicillin allergic, what would be the recommendation for antibiotic prophylaxis?**

Trimethoprim-sulfamethoxazole PLUS clindamycin.

❏❏ **Protective measures that might be recommended for an athlete about to run a cross country race in a wooded area on Eastern Long Island to prevent tick bites might include:**

Tucking pant legs into socks, applying permethrin to clothing to decrease tick attachment, applying DEET to the skin and inspecting exposed areas after outdoor exposure for attached ticks.

❏❏ **T/F: If after an outdoor exposure as in the previous question, a tick is found attached to the lower extremity, vaseline should be applied over the area before attempting removal of the tick.**

False.

❏❏ **T/F: If a tick is found on the athlete's skin after a sporting event in an area endemic for Lyme disease prophylactic treatment with amoxicillin is indicated to prevent subsequent development of Lyme disease.**

False.

❏❏ **A cross country runner, who had a splenectomy 3 years ago secondary to trauma, develops high fever, malaise and hepatomegaly 2 weeks after participating in a meet in a wooded area of Eastern Connecticut. What is the most likely diagnosis?**

Babesiosis.

❏❏ **How is this condition diagnosed?**

Giemsa- or Wright-stained blood smear (thick or thin smears).
Or Serologic testing for detection of Babesia antibodies.

❏❏ **What does the antimicrobial therapy for this condition consists of?**

Atovaquone and azithromycin or clindamycin and quinine for 7 to 10 days.

❏❏ **Two to three hours after a post-game buffet of Chinese food, 16 of 25 members of an athletic team develop the acute onset of nausea, vomiting and abdominal cramps. What is the most likely cause of this outbreak?**

Food poisoning with toxin of *Bacillus cereus*; most commonly associated with fried rice.

❏❏ **Over a 7-day period after eating together in a fast food restaurant, a number of members of an athletic team develop bloody diarrhea. Laboratory testing confirms a diagnosis confirms a diagnosis of *E. coliO157:H7*. What would be the most appropriate antibiotic therapy for symptomatic individuals?**

None; Trimethoprim-sulfamethoxazole may increase risk of hemolytic uremic syndrome.

❏❏ **T/F: A student athlete recovering from Salmonella gastroenteritis should not be allowed to return to competitive athletics until he has a documented negative stool culture.**

False.

❏❏ **T/F: A student athlete, diagnosed with Shigella gastroenteritis may return to the team once his/her symptoms have resolved regardless of stool culture results.**

False.

❏❏ **T/F Outbreaks of adenoviral pharyngoconjunctival fever have been associated with inadequate chlorination of swimming pools.**

True.

❏❏ **T/F: Students competing in athletics should be screened for HIV, Hepatitis B and Hepatitis C prior to joining a team in order to prevent transmission to other students.**

False.

❏❏ **T/F: Athletes infected with HIV, Hepatitis B virus or Hepatitis C virus should not be allowed to participate in select competitive sports.**

False.

❏❏ **T/F: The team physician should be aware of any HIV-positive athletes on a team in case an injury with active bleeding occurs.**

False.

❏❏ **T/F: Staff caring for an athlete with a bleeding injury should wear gloves (vinyl or latex) and employ good hand washing technique regardless of the athlete's HIV status.**

True.

☐☐ **T/F: In the absence of available gloves if an athlete suffers a bleeding injury, a towel should be used to cover the wound until proper barrier protection and technique can be applied.**

True.

☐☐ **T/F Mouth-to-mouth resuscitation is only recommended only if Ambu bags and oral airways are not available to prevent potential transmission of pathogens.**

True.

☐☐ **T/F: Athletes with tinea pedis should be exclude from swimming pools and walking barefoot in locker rooms and shower areas until treatment has been initiated.**

True.

☐☐ **An athlete diagnosed with Group A streptococcal pharyngitis may return to school _____ after initiation of antibiotic therapy.**

24 hours.

☐☐ **An athlete with 2 weeks of cough is diagnosed with pertussis. He may safely return to school _____ after initiation of antimicrobial therapy.**

5 days.

☐☐ **What is the drug of choice for treatment of pertussis?**

Erythromycin.

☐☐ **T/F: All teammates of the athlete with pertussis should receive antimicrobial prophylaxis.**

False.

☐☐ **T/F: All teammates of the athlete with pertussis who do not have a documented history of a complete series of pertussis immunization should receive a booster dose of pertussis vaccine in this setting.**

False.

☐☐ **T/F: Routine annual influenza vaccine should be considered for members of athletic teams.**

True.

❏❏ **T/F: If there is a documented outbreak of Influenza B among members of an athletic team, chemoprophylaxis with amantadine may protect uninfected teammates from illness.**

False; the newer approved neuraminidase inhibitor, Oseltamivir (Tamiflu) may be effective for prophylaxis against Influenza types A and B; amantadine is only effective against type A strains.

❏❏ **T/F: Meningococcal vaccine should be considered for all incoming college freshman athletes who will be living in dormitories.**

True.

❏❏ **T/F: Pneumococcal polysaccharide or pneumococcal conjugate vaccine should be considered for all incoming college freshman athletes who will be living in dormitories.**

False.

❏❏ **An athlete is diagnosed with Hepatitis A infection. How long should he/she be excluded from school?**

One week after onset of the illness and until clinically well enough to return.

❏❏ **T/F: Teammates of an individual with Hepatitis A who eat in the same dining facility should receive immunoglobulin (IG) within two weeks of exposure to the infected individual.**

True.

❏❏ **A school athletic team is invited to participate in a school tournament in Canada. Pre-travel advice includes recommendation for Hepatitis A prophylaxis. How is this accomplished?**

Immunoglobulin or 2 doses Hepatitis A vaccine (with 6 months between the 2 doses of vaccine).

❏❏ **T/F: A wrestler diagnosed with impetigo may safely return to competition after 24 hours of antimicrobial therapy.**

True.

❏❏ **T/F: Tinea capitis may be spread in locker rooms by sharing combs, hair brushes or hair ornaments.**

True.

❏❏ **T/F: Due to a documented increased risk among student athletes, annual tuberculin skin testing (PPD) is recommended for these individuals.**

False.

SPECIAL CONSIDERATION

ENVIRONMENTAL CONCERNS

❏❏ **What physical sign is the best predictor of early high altitude cerebral edema (HACE)?**

Ataxia.

❏❏ **What is the most common form of altitude illness? What percentage of travelers will experience this?**

Acute mountain sickness (AMS). 20-30% of those rapidly traveling to 8,000 to 9,000 feet.

❏❏ **Name a key physiological response to hypobaric hypoxia. What is the limiting factor to this response?**

The hypoxic ventilatory response. This response, mediated by the carotid body and the central respiratory center, is limited by the resultant respiratory alkalosis. Excretion of bicarbonate by the kidneys gradually allows further increases in ventilation and acclimatization.

❏❏ **What is the best way to prevent all forms of altitude illness?**

Graded ascent. Maximum of 3000 meters initially and maximum of 600-900 meters/day or "climb high, sleep low".

❏❏ **What are the earliest symptoms of high altitude pulmonary edema (HAPE)? What pharmacologic therapy is most useful for the treatment of HAPE?**

Decreased exercise tolerance and increased recovery time from exercise. Nifedipine.

❏❏ **A diet high in carbohydrates started one to two days prior to ascent can decrease the incidence of this illness by 30 per cent at altitudes greater than 16,000 feet.**

Acute mountain sickness (AMS).

❏❏ **What is the most accurate method for measuring environmental heat stress? Why?**

The wet-bulb globe thermometer (WBGT). The WBGT accounts for the effects of radiant heat and humidity as well as the ambient temperature.

❑❑ **What is the primary cause of heat cramps? How is it treated?**

Salt depletion. It is treated with salt supplementation, fluid replacement, resting in a cool environment and gentle stretching of involved muscles.

❑❑ **Describe the beneficial changes in sweat and urine that occur after 1-2 weeks of heat stress that promote acclimatization. What is the mediator?**

Acclimatization changes include earlier onset of sweating, higher volume of sweating, and decreased sodium concentration in sweat and urine. It is mediated by aldosterone.

❑❑ **Class of drugs that most often cause impaired sweating and heat illness.**

Anticholinergics.

❑❑ **What are the classic symptoms of heat stroke? Which of these is the least reliable?**

Severe hyperthermia, CNS disturbance, and cessation of sweating. Each of these findings may be problematic but cessation of sweating is the least reliable and usually occurs very late in the illness.

❑❑ **What is the most ominous prognostic sign in patients suffering from heatstroke?**

Hypotension.

❑❑ **What physiologic difference makes children less susceptible to salt depletion during heat or exercise?**

Decreased sweat volume and decreased salt concentration in the sweat of children.

❑❑ **Is lightning most like direct current (DC) or alternating current (AC)?**

DC. However, it has been best described as a unidirectional massive current impulse.

❑❑ **What is the most common initial cardiac dysrhythmia after lightning injury?**

Asystole.

❑❑ **The most common symptoms of a victim of unwitnessed mild lightning injury?**

Confusion and amnesia.

❑❑ **Following a lightning injury prolonged resuscitation may be necessary due to prolonged paralysis of this organ system.**

The respiratory system. Cardiac activity may return long before respiration.

❏❏ **First and second-degree burns over much of the body are present after this most common mechanism of lightning injury.**

Flashover phenomenon (also called arborescent burns).

❏❏ **Form of solar radiation with fairly constant intensity throughout the day.**

UVA.

❏❏ **Name two adaptive responses of the skin to chronic exposure to ultraviolet radiation.**

Melanogenesis and thickening of the stratum corneum.

❏❏ **Form of solar radiation responsible for 98-99% of *delayed* skin erythema after sun exposure.**

UVB.

❏❏ **What is the most common adverse reaction to PABA containing sunscreens?**

Contact or photocontact dermatitis. In addition, it's UVB absorption peak at 296nm is relatively far from the UVB-induced erythema peak at 307nm.

❏❏ **What is the maximum recommended weight of a backpack for children?**

20% of the child's body weight.

❏❏ **What complication has been reported with the use of DEET in children and what is the maximum concentration recommended for children?**

Toxic encephalopathy. 35% maximum concentration.

❏❏ **Name the safest drugs for the prevention of malaria in children less than 15 kg.**

Chloroquine (Aralen) and Proguanil (Paludrine).

❏❏ **Name four identifying characteristics of snakes of the crotalidae family (pit vipers).**

Facial pits, vertical elliptical pupils, triangular head distinct from the remainder of the body and a single row of subcaudate scutes or scales.

❏❏ **What are the three most important steps in assisting the victim of a venomous snakebite?**

Keep victim calm. Immobilize bitten extremity. Seek medical attention.

❏❏ **Name the organism responsible for Lyme disease and the most common insect vector.**

Borrelia burgdorferi and Ixodes scapularis (dammini).

❏❏ **What is the most common skin manifestation of early Lyme disease and what percentage of patients will manifest this condition?**

Erythema chronicum migrans. 60%-80%.

❏❏ **Type IV (delayed hypersensitivity) reaction occurs most frequently after exposure to this non-volatile oil. What percentage of the population is susceptible?**

Urushiol. Approximately 50%.

❏❏ **Name five groups of toxic chemicals found in plants.**

Alkaloids, Glycosides, Resins, Oxalates, and Phytotoxins.

❏❏ **Patients with delayed symptoms (4 or more hours) of toxicity following toxic mushroom ingestion are more likely to have ingested mushrooms from which genera?**

Amanita or Gyromitra.

❏❏ **What is the name of the regularly updated and authoritative source of information on travel medicine?**

The CDC's "Health Information for International Travel" ("the yellow book").

❏❏ **What is the mechanism of arterial gas embolism in scuba divers?**

Entry of air into the pulmonary capillaries via ruptured alveoli.

❏❏ **What is the most common form of barotrauma in divers?**

External ear squeeze (sometimes called middle ear squeeze).

❏❏ **How does decompression sickness in divers occur and what law of physics is responsible for this problem?**

Rapid ascent while diving causes the formation of nitrogen gas bubbles in the tissue and in venous blood. Henry's law states that the amount of gas dissolved in a liquid at a given temperature is a function of the partial pressure of the gas in contact with the liquid and the solubility coefficient of the gas.

❏❏ **What is the recommended surface interval after scuba diving before air travel should occur?**

A minimum of 12 hours after the last dive. 24 hours or more should be considered for divers who have made multiple dives for several days.

☐☐ **The Heimlich maneuver should only be performed on drowning victims in the following circumstance.**

When CPR or ventilation fails due to suspected blockage of the airway with foreign matter.

☐☐ **This substance, when lost or diluted in a drowning victim, may lead to atelectasis, V/Q mismatch and breakdown of alveolar capillary membrane.**

Surfactant.

☐☐ **What common injury in white water kayakers is associated with a maneuver called the high brace?**

Anterior shoulder dislocation.

☐☐ **This salt-water coelenterate can cause envenomation associated with high mortality. What is its common and scientific name?**

The box jellyfish. Chironex fleckeri.

☐☐ **What is the best first-aid for victims of jellyfish stings? Venomous fish stings?**

5% Acetic acid rinse. Prolonged hot water immersion.

☐☐ **This potentially fatal problem may occur with rough handling of the victim or with chest compressions in a victim of severe hypothermia.**

Ventricular fibrillation.

☐☐ **What is the classic ECG finding in hypothermic patients?**

Osborne waves.

☐☐ **Victims of more than 30 minutes of cold water submersion have survived only when this form of treatment is available.**

Advanced life support.

☐☐ **Once initiated, resuscitation should continue in victims of cold water submersion until the core temperature reaches this temperature.**

86°F (30°C).

☐☐ **What is the name of the phenomenon of continued drop in core body temperature after rescue that may occur in victims of *acute* hypothermia?**

After drop.

❏❏ **What physical finding indicates a hypothermia victim has progressed beyond mild hypothermia?**

The absence of shivering.

❏❏ **This cold weather, non-freezing injury results from prolonged exposure of the foot to a cold, wet environment.**

Trenchfoot.

❏❏ **What is the best treatment for severe frostbite?**

Immersion of frozen part in 104°-108°F water.

❏❏ **Name the eye problem caused by prolonged exposure to UVB radiation. What percentage of UVB is reflected by snow?**

Snow blindness. 85%.

PSYCHOSOCIAL ASPECTS OF SPORTS PARTICIPATION

❑❑ **What are a few of the tests used to determine athlete's personality?**

The State Trait Anxiety Inventory, the test of attention and interpersonal style, the profile of mood states, the Eyseneck Personality Inventory.

❑❑ **What are the five guidelines to build motivation?**

Both situations and traits motivate people; people have multiple motives for involvement; change the environment to enhance motivation; leaders influence motivation; behavior modification or change undesirable participant motives.

❑❑ **What are the three views of motivation?**

Participant centered, situation centered and interactional orientation.

❑❑ **What are the important psychological skills that can help facilitate an athlete's ability to cope with injury rehabilitation?**

Interpersonal Communication, positive reinforcement, continued team involvement, realistic goal setting.

❑❑ **What are the organizations for American Sport and Exercise Psychology?**

Association for the Advancement of Applied Sport Psychology, American Psychological Association (APA) Division 47- Sport and Exercise Psychology, North American Society for the Psychology of Sport and Physical Activity (NASPSPA).

❑❑ **What is the difference between outcome goal orientation and task goal orientation?**

Outcome orientation focuses on comparing performance with and defeating others and task goal orientation focuses on comparing with your own performance.

❑❑ **What are the problems with outcome orientations?**

People will have difficulties maintaining high-perceived competence and may demonstrate a maladaptive behavioral pattern.

❑❑ **What are the best ways to prevent maladaptive tendencies?**

Help athletes set task goals and downplay outcome goals.

☐☐ **What is the one thing an instructor should not do when giving feedback to an athlete?**

Attribute success to luck.

☐☐ **What is one of the key attributions an instructor can use with an athlete?**

Emphasize mastery goal by focusing on individual improvement.

☐☐ **What are three important areas of emotion that sports psychologists study?**

Arousal, stress and anxiety.

☐☐ **What is arousal?**

Arousal is a general physiological and psychological activation of the person that varies on a continuum from deep sleep to intense excitement.

☐☐ **What are the two components of anxiety?**

State anxiety - that which apples to the emotional and Trait anxiety – that which is part of the personality.

☐☐ **Is there a relationship between state and trait anxiety?**

Yes. There is a direct relationship between a person's level of state anxiety and their trait anxiety.

☐☐ **What is the definition of stress?**

Stress is a " substantial imbalance between demand (physical or psychological) and response capability where failure to meet that demand has important consequences."

☐☐ **What are 4 inter related stages of stress?**

Environmental demand, Perception of demands, Stress response, Behavioral consequences.

☐☐ **What is the facilitation theory?**

It is the theory that an audience creates arousal in a performer, which impairs performance on difficult tasks that are unlearned and improves performance on tasks that are well known.

☐☐ **Describe the inverted U hypothesis regarding arousal states and performance.**

High performance occurs at an optimal level of arousal; lesser performance will occur at either very low or very high arousal.

☐☐ **How does increase arousal affect performance?**

Increased arousal may cause increased muscle tension and coordination difficulties and it may cause changes in attention and concentration.

"Basketball is a sport in which success, as symbolized by the championship, requires that the community goal prevail over selfish impulses.... The less conflict there is off court, the more the inevitable friction can be minimized...teams develop when talents and personalities mesh." Bill Bradley

❏❏ **Which is the approach used by sports psychologists to study competition?**

Social evaluation approach.

❏❏ **What is the subjective situation an athlete may use to evaluate how well they compete?**

Perceived ability, motivation, importance of the competitive situation.

❏❏ **What modifications can be made to change the perception of success or failure in a sport?**

Lower the basket in basketball; use smaller balls for basketball, volleyball or football; do not keep official score, allow player to stay at bat until the ball is hit into fair territory and rotate positions on the team.

❏❏ **Are there cross-cultural differences in competitive orientation?**

Yes, cultures differ in fostering competitive attitudes.

❏❏ **What is Orlick's basic philosophy of competitive games?**

Competition and cooperation are complementary. Most activities can be classified into one of five categories: Competitive means – competitive ends, Cooperative means – competitive ends, Individual means – individual ends, Cooperative means – individual ends and Cooperative means – cooperative ends.

❏❏ **Does competition produce negative consequences?**

No. It is the emphasis on winning, which may be counterproductive.

❏❏ **What are the two basic premises that underlie reinforcing behavior?**

Positive reinforcement (good consequences following a certain behavior) which increases the chance of wanted behaviors and negative reinforcement (unpleasant consequences follow a certain behavior) which should lead to a reduction of undesirable behavior.

❏❏ **What are a few negative results from negative reinforcement?**

A fear of failure can be created which leads to an athlete who may " choke " under pressure, players may be tentative rather than take the risks if they are concerned that they may be pulled from a game, unintentional reinforcement of uninvited behavior by paying attention to it, creation of an unpleasant atmosphere where the coach is resented.

❐❐ **What is an effective way to choose effective positive reinforcers?**

Know the likes and dislikes of the people you work with.

❐❐ **What are material reinforcers of good behavior?**

Trophies, ribbons, medals, T-shirts.

❐❐ **Many coaches / teachers reward outcomes of a performance. What are other behaviors that could be rewarded?**

Behaviors to be rewarded are successful approximations, performance (not outcome), effort and emotional and social skills.

❐❐ **What percentage of reinforcement should be positive?**

Researchers say the 80 – 90 % of reinforcement should be positive.

❐❐ **What are four important guidelines for giving negative feedback?**

Address the behavior not the person, do not use physical activity as a punishment, impose negative feedback impersonally (do not yell), do not give negative feedback while an athlete is playing, do not embarrass individuals in front of teammates.

❐❐ **What is a behavioral program?**

The systematic application of the basic principles of positive and negative reinforcement.

❐❐ **How can a behavioral program be implemented for a team?**

First, a few specific behaviors need to be worked with and defined. Then the behaviors should be recorded and meaningful feedback given. The outcomes that need to be changed should be clear to the athlete and a reward system needs to be tailored to the specific athletes.

❐❐ **What are intrinsic motivators?**

Those who are intrinsically motivated strive internally to be competent and compete for the joy of the sport. They want to learn skills to the best of their ability.

❐❐ **External rewards have negative impact on intrinsic rewards. What is the negative impact?**

Rewards that are controlling the reason for their behavior is beyond the sport (money); rewards that are based on information regarding competence may only serve to decrease feelings of competence in the person who does not receive it.

❑❑ What are 5 ways to increase intrinsic motivation?

Provide successful experiences, give rewards contingent on performance, vary content of performance drills, set realistic goals, and allow athletes to take responsibility in making the rules.

❑❑ Flow is important in intrinsic motivation. What are factors which disrupt flow in an athlete?

Physical problems and mistakes, inability to maintain focus, negative mental attitude.

❑❑ What are the 4 stages of development that a team must go through to change from a collection of individuals to a team?

Forming, storming, norming and performing.

❑❑ What is forming, storming, norming and performing?

Forming – interpersonal relationships are created; *storming* – rebellion, infighting and interpersonal conflict; *norming* – hostility replaced by solidarity and cooperation; *performing* – team members band together to channel their energies for team success.

❑❑ What is Steiner's model of productivity for an athletic team?

Actual productivity = potential productivity - losses due to faulty group processes.

❑❑ What are the faulty group processes that can detract from a group's overall productivity?

Motivation losses (when all of the athletes are not giving 100%) and coordination losses (when timing between the athletes is off or unproductive strategies are used).

❑❑ What is social loafing?

When individuals within a group or team give less than 100 % of effort.

❑❑ What are the three principles to help build unity within a group?

Increase identifiability within a team, conduct individual meetings, and incorporate low intensity practices/ drills into the season.

❑❑ What are two forces that keep members in a group?

Attractiveness of the group and the benefits an athlete can achieve by being associated with a group.

❑❑ What are two kinds of measures to gauge cohesion?

Questionnaires, in particular the Multidimensional Sports Cohesion Instrument and sociograms.

❑❑ **What is a sociogram?**

It is a tool to measure social cohesion. It discloses affiliation and attraction among group members, and may demonstrate cliques, social isolation and members' perception of group cohesiveness.

❑❑ **Although much research has been done on cohesion and performance, what are other factors that are associated with cohesion?**

Team satisfaction, conformity, stability, group goals and adherence to exercise.

❑❑ **What are barriers to group cohesion?**

Personality clashes, conflict of social roles, power struggles, frequent turnovers and disagreement on group goals and objectives.

❑❑ **If you were on a team what would you do to build team cohesion?**

Get to know teammates, help other members of the team whenever possible, give peers positive reinforcement, be responsible, communicate honestly and openly with the coach, resolve conflicts as soon as possible, give 100 % and give it 100 % of the time.

❑❑ **Does cohesion lead to winning or does winning lead to cohesion?**

There is data to support the relationship between early season performance and later cohesion, but not visa versa.

❑❑ **What is the difference between a manager and a leader?**

A manager takes care of scheduling, budgeting and organizing and a leader deals more with goals and objectives and direction of a team.

❑❑ **What are three useful components of an effective team leader?**

Excellent communication, knowledgeable instruction and demonstration and responses to behaviors which are reactive or spontaneous.

❑❑ **What is the difference between mistake-contingent encouragement and mistake- contingent technical instruction?**

Mistake contingent encouragement is encouragement given to a player following a mistake and mistake contingent technical instruction is showing an athlete how to fix their mistake.

❑❑ **What is the Multidimensional Model of Leadership?**

It is the theory which shows that sport leaders exhibit three types of behaviors: required, preferred and actual. Required are those which are demanded of the leader; preferred, which reflects more of what the group wants and; actual which are affected directly by the personality, ability and experience.

❑❑ **Describe the four components of effective leadership.**

Leader's qualities, leadership style, situational factors and member characteristics.

❑❑ **What are three guideline coaches may use for consistency in communication?**

Never miss an opportunity to praise an athlete; maintain an open door policy and be sincere about it; show the same compassion on the field as you do in the office.

❑❑ **Define active listening.**

Pay attention to content of what the speaker is saying, acknowledge and respond to the message and give appropriate feedback.

❑❑ **What is the sandwich technique for giving criticism?**

Three sequential elements should be followed: first give a positive statement; followed by future oriented instructions and ending with a positive statement.

❑❑ **What is PST?**

PST is Psychological Skills Training.

❑❑ **State three reasons why PST is important.**

Knowledge of PST can help coaches deal with the athlete who can't perform during a game, who is depressed because they are not recovering from an injury quickly enough or experience a lack of motivation to exercise.

❑❑ **Is there any empiric evidence that PST improves sports performance?**

Yes. Psychological skills development such as developing competitive plans, daily training goals, simulations in practice, building confidence, task oriented thoughts, positive imagery and overcoming obstacles have been shown to enhance performance.

❑❑ **What are techniques that have been shown to be effective in reducing anxiety in the athlete?**

Progressive muscle relaxation, breath control, systemic desensitization and biofeedback.

❑❑ **What is cognitive- affective stress management training?**

It is a comprehensive skills program designed to help teach an athlete integrated coping responses. It uses relaxation and cognitive components to help control emotional responses.

❑❑ **What are 4 uses of imagery?**

Improve concentration, build confidence, help deal with injury, and control emotional responses.

❑❑ **Discuss the relationship between confidence and performance.**

It is an inverted U relationship; performance improves to an optimal level of confidence. Beyond this, overconfidence will lead to a performance that will suffer.

❑❑ **What is the role of psychological factors in athletic injuries?**

Research has shown that there is a relationship between life stress and injury in the athlete. This may be due to attentional disruption and / or increased muscle tension.

❑❑ **Is there a relationship between coaches who ask for 110 % and increased injuries?**

Yes. Coaches that convey winning above all and a " no pain, no gain " attitude may actually be setting their athletes up for an injury.

❑❑ **How can sports psychology facilitate injury treatment and rehabilitation?**

By building rapport with the athlete, the athlete can be taught specific psychological coping skills (goal setting, positive self talk), prepare them to deal with setback and foster social support.

❑❑ **What are risk factors for developing an eating disorder?**

Pressure and desire to optimize performance at a lower weight, perfectionism, compulsiveness and high achievement expectations.

❑❑ **What are 4 diagnostic criteria for anorexia nervosa?**

Refusal to maintain body weight leading to a body weight less than 85% of expected weight, intense fear of gaining weight, disturbance in the ways one's body is perceived, amenorrhea in post menarchal females (absence of at least 3 menstrual cycles).

❑❑ **What are 4 diagnostic criteria for bulimia nervosa?**

Recurrent episodes of binge eating, recurrent inappropriate compensatory behavior to prevent weight gain, binge eating/compensatory behavior occurs at least twice a week for three months, self evaluation unduly influenced by weight.

❑❑ **What are the four characteristics of burnout?**

Loss of desire to play, lack of caring, sleep disturbance, headaches, mood changes, substance abuse, emotional isolation, increase anxiety, physical and mental exhaustion.

❑❑ **Describe three techniques to reduce burnout.**

Set short term goals for competition and practice; express feelings in a constructive manner; and manage post competition emotions.

☐☐ **What are factors associated with burnout in young athletes?**

Overtraining, high self-expectations, " win at all costs " attitude, parental pressure, long repetitive practices, inconsistent coaching practices, overuse injuries and excessive time demands.

☐☐ **Describe the four criteria for aggression.**

Aggression is a behavior, which involves harm or injury. It is directed to a living being and involves intent.

☐☐ **What are 4 important theories in sport psychology about the origin of aggression?**

Instinct theory – the innate instinct to be aggressive; Frustration – aggression theory – where a frustration naturally leads to aggressive behavior; Social learning theory – aggression is learned from others and the Revised Frustration – aggression theory which combines the original frustration aggression model with the social learning theory. This theory states that although frustration does not always lead to aggression, it increases the likelihood by increasing anger and arousal.

☐☐ **What is Eccles' model of achievement?**

Eccles found, through her research, that gender differences in expectations for sports participation do not suddenly appear, but develop over time. She found that activity choice depended on socialization differences in boys and girls.

☐☐ **What is Title IX?**

Title IX, passed in 1972, states that no persons in the United States shall, on the basis of sex, be excluded from participation in any activity receiving federal funding.

☐☐ **Since the passing of Title IX, what has happened to coaching of women's teams?**

Women coaching women's teams has dropped from 90 to 48%.

PROCEDURES

CARDIOPULMONARY RESUSCITATION

❑❑ **What is the basis for the recommendation to activate the 911-EMS system as the initial step in adult cardiopulmonary arrest?**

This recommendation is based on the high frequency of ventricular fibrillation in this population. The goal is to get the defibrillator to the patient as soon as possible.

❑❑ **Primary confirmation of correct endotracheal tube placement includes:**

Visualization of the tube through the cords.
5 point auscultation.
Bilateral chest expansion.
Condensation in the tube.

❑❑ **What is the basis for the recommendation for smaller tidal volumes during rescue breathing?**

Smaller tidal volumes will decrease the amount of gastric distention and its complications.

❑❑ **T/F: In pediatric resuscitations the intraosseous technique is acceptable and recommended in pediatric victims including children over the age of 6 years.**

True. The intraosseous technique is acceptable and recommended in pediatric victims, including children over age 6 years.

❑❑ **Name 4 potential airway emergencies that may occur in the artificially ventilated patient.**

Displacement of the endotracheal tube.
Obstruction of the endotracheal tube.
Pneumothorax.
Equipment failure.

❑❑ **In which direction would you expect the oxyhemoglobin desaturation curve to shift in a patient with metabolic acidosis undergoing resuscitation?**

Acidosis shifts the oxyhemoglobin curve to the right.

❏❏ **T/F: Vasopressin is equivalent to epinephrine for refractory ventricular fibrillation and pulseless ventricular tachycardia.**

True. Vasopressin is equivalent to epinephrine for refractory ventricular fibrillation and pulseless ventricular tachycardia.

❏❏ **What is the most common cause of airway obstruction in the unconscious patient?**

The tongue and mandibular soft tissue.

❏❏ **What is the most likely cause of death in commotio cordis?**

Lethal ventricular arrhythmia.

❏❏ **What is the most common condition associated with "sudden death " in the adult athlete?**

Hypertrophic cardiac myopathy.

❏❏ **What does the combination of hypertension and bradycardia suggest in the unconscious athlete who has sustained a severe head/ neck injury?**

Increasing intracranial pressure.

❏❏ **What would you expect to see in the vital signs of an athlete with a cervical spine fracture/dislocation and spinal shock?**

Bradycardia and hypotension.

❏❏ **T/F: Anaphylactic shock generally develops over 6 - 8 hours.**

False. Shock associated with anaphylaxis may develop quickly.

❏❏ **Name 6 of the possible causes of pulseless electrical activity that can occur in the athlete.**

Hypovolemia.
Hypoxia.
Cardiac tamponade.
Hypothermia.
Acidosis.
Tension pneumothorax.

❏❏ **T/F: Automated External Defibrillators (AED) are recommended for use only by physicians licensed to practice medicine in the particular state.**

International Guidelines 2000 recommends that all trained responders be prepared to use an AED.

❏❏ **What is the recommended rate of chest compressions for adult resuscitation?**

100 compressions per minute. This recommendation is for both health professionals and lay rescuers and should be used with both 1 and 2 person rescuers.

❏❏ **T/F: Laryngeal Mask Airways (LMA) are an acceptable method for securing the airway in an unconscious adult victim.**

True. The LMA is an acceptable technique for securing the airway in an unconscious adult victim.

❏❏ **What is the most effective dosing schedule for epinephrine in the case of an adult patient with pulseless ventricular tachycardia?**

Epinephrine 1 mg every 3 - 5 minutes is recommended.

❏❏ **T/F: Following resuscitative efforts on the playing field, patients who are mildly hypothermic should be aggressively rewarmed.**

False. Active rewarming of the mildly hypothermic patient who has undergone cardiopulmonary resuscitation is not recommended.

❏❏ **T/F: In adults, resuscitation medications which are given by endotracheal tube should be administered at the same doses as when given intravenously.**

False. In adults the doses of epinephrine, atropine and lidocaine should be 2 - 2.5 times the intravenous dose when administered via the endotracheal tube.

❏❏ **Under which circumstance might the end tidal CO_2 monitor give falsely low values?**

Falsely low values may be seen in the patient with asystole even when the endotracheal tube is in the trachea.

❏❏ **What is the correct initial compression-ventilation ratio for adult CPR victims?**

A compression to ventilation ratio of 15: 2 is recommended until the airway has been secured.

❏❏ **Under which circumstance would you consider hyperventilation in the postresuscitative care of an athlete?**

When there are signs of cerebral herniation after resuscitation.

❏❏ **What are the drugs of choice in stable wide complex ventricular tachycardia?**

Amiodarone and sotalol are first line drugs for stable wide complex ventricular tachycardia.

❑❑ **What is the first pharmacologic intervention indicated for symptomatic bradycardia?**

Atropine.

❑❑ **What is the leading cause of death and disability in the pediatric age group?**

Trauma.

❑❑ **What type of oxygen mask can deliver inspired oxygen concentrations of 95%?**

Properly fit nonrebreathing masks with an oxygen flow rate of 10 - 12 L/minute.

❑❑ **List potential complications of intraosseous infusions?**

Tibial fracture.
Compartment syndrome.
Skin necrosis.
Osteomyelitis.

❑❑ **The pulse oximeter is a useful adjunct in resuscitation because the percent oxygen saturation has a linear relationship with the PO_2.**

False. The sigmoid shape of the oxyhemoglobin saturation curve demonstrates that the relationship is nonlinear.

❑❑ **List 4 frequent resuscitation scenarios in which the pulse oximeter would be unreliable.**

Vasoconstriction.
Hypotension.
Hypothermia.
Severe anemia.

❑❑ **What special precaution is mandatory during the resuscitation of the athlete who has sustained a head injury on the playing field?**

Cervical spine immobilization.

❑❑ **List 2 methods that may be employed to establish an emergency surgical airway in an athlete who has sustained a serious maxillofacial trauma and requires airway maintenance.**

Needle cricothyroidotomy with jet insufflation.
Surgical cricothyroidotomy.

❑❑ **What is the maximum concentration of inspired oxygen that can be administered with standard mouth to mouth resuscitation?**

A maximum concentration of 16 - 17 % can be obtained.

❏❏ **List clinical signs that would alert you to a diagnosis of a tension pneumothorax?**

Severe respiratory distress.
Hyperresonance to percussion.
Diminished breath sound on the affected side.
Deviation of the trachea and mediastinum away from the affected side.

❏❏ **What is the major risk of administering a high infusion rate of dopamine (> 20mcg/kg/minute) in a pediatric aged athlete with shock?**

Severe peripheral vasoconstriction and ischemia.

❏❏ **T/F: Hypotension is an early indicator of impending hypovolemic shock in children with trauma.**

False. Delayed capillary refill is an early indicator of poor perfusion. Hypotension occurs when the child has lost at least 25 - 30 % of their blood volume.

❏❏ **Which blood type is considered the universal donor?**

Type O negative blood.

❏❏ **What are the two most likely chest injuries to impede initial stabilization of the pediatric aged athlete?**

Tension pneumothorax and open pneumothorax.

❏❏ **How are tension pneumothoraces treated?**

Tension pneumothorax is a life threatening chest injury. Urgent decompression is required with needle decompression followed by the placement of a chest tube.

❏❏ **Does the Good Samaritan law protect team physicians from liability while engaged in an onfield resuscitation of a participating athlete?**

No. The Good Samaritan legislation was designed to protect lay persons and now in some jurisdictions health care providers who do not have a "duty to respond" and who are "acting in good faith".

PROCEDURES

EXERCISE TESTING

❏❏ **List the standard physiological measurements monitored during a cardiopulmonary exercise study.**

Heart rate, blood pressure, oxygen consumption, CO_2 production and ventilation.

❏❏ **List four physiological mechanisms which can be responsible for a fall in Oxygen saturation during exercise.**

Right to left shunt.
V/Q mismatch.
O_2 diffusion abnormality.
Low F_IO_2 (altitude).

❏❏ **T/F: Minute ventilation during exercise will increase only by increases in tidal volume.**

False. Minute ventilation can increase by increasing either tidal volume, respiratory rate or both.

❏❏ **The ratio of maximum ventilation divided by maximal voluntary ventilation (VE/MVV) would help describe what type of limitation to exercise?**

Lung limitations.

❏❏ **Cardiac output increases during exercise. Cardiac output increases during early exercise with increases primarily in this variable.**

Stroke volume.

❏❏ **Cardiac output during heavy exercise (above the ventilatory anaerobic threshold) increases primarily by increases in this variable?**

Heart rate.

❏❏ **T/F: Stroke volume will increase more during supine exercise than upright exercise.**

False. Stroke volume is maximized at rest in the supine position.

❏❏ **During exercise the pulmonary vascular resistance (PVR) will change. What change occurs and why?**

Vasodilatation of the pulmonary vascular bed and increased recruitment of circulation causes the PVR to fall.

❏❏ **T/F: Mixed venous O₂ tension (P$_V$O$_2$) increases during exercise.**

False. It will fall with an increase in oxygen consumption.

❏❏ **What event is best described as a positive response to an exercise challenge in an asthmatic athlete?**

Acute bronchoconstriction.

❏❏ **What common theory (protocol) is assumed when performing an exercise challenge for asthma?**

Airway drying and cooling using a high load, steady state exercise protocol.

❏❏ **T/F: Resting lung function (vital capacity, FEV$_1$ and DLCO) can predict exercise capacity (VO$_2$ max) in normal children.**

False. Lung volumes do not predict exercise capacity.

❏❏ **During exercise the breakpoint for the anaerobic threshold by ventilatory parameters is where what 4 variables change and in what direction do they change?**

Minute ventilation increases.
End tidal CO$_2$ falls.
Ventilatory equivalents for O$_2$ and CO$_2$ increase.

❏❏ **An increase in diastolic blood pressure best represents what hemodynamic event?**

Fall in cardiac output, which causes acute vasoconstriction.

❏❏ **Measurements of arterial and venous lactic acid help to determine what exercise phenomena?**

The anaerobic threshold.

❏❏ **Pulmonary transit time refers to what physiologic process?**

How long the red blood cell is in the pulmonary circuit to become oxygenated.

❏❏ **When exercising a subject with lung disease, the determination of the PA-a CO$_2$ gradient would indicate?**

CO$_2$ retention.

❑❑ **T/F: During exercise the changes in ventilation mirror the changes in end tidal CO₂ (P_ETCO₂).**

False. P_ETCO₂ increase slightly and falls at the onset of anaerobic metabolism.

❑❑ **T/F: During exercise the changes in cardiac output have a similar increase to changes in systolic blood pressure.**

True. Increases in systolic blood pressure will mirror changes in cardiac output.

❑❑ **T/F: Diastolic blood pressure will increase in proportion to increases in external work?**

False. Diastolic blood pressure remains unchanged throughout an exercise test.

❑❑ **List two differences between exercise on a bicycle ergometer and a motorized treadmill.**

Cycle ergometry is more muscle specific to the leg muscles leading to earlier fatigue relative to heart rate. Treadmill exercise is body weight dependent and may be more difficult for large and/or obese patients.

❑❑ **T/F: Anaerobic exercise requires less O₂ and can be sustained for less time than aerobic exercise.**

True. Anaerobic exercise will only last 30 – 90 seconds; aerobic exercise can last for several hours depending upon level of intensity.

❑❑ **T/F: An exercise prescription can be written from the results of a submaximal stress test.**

True. Often this is the sole purpose of performing a submaximal stress test in a healthy population.

❑❑ **T/F: The energy cost for any specific submaximal workload on a cycle ergometer is approximately the same for any individual with normal body weight.**

True. Cycle ergometry is body weight independent and the energy cost will be determined by the workload.

❑❑ **Oxygen consumption can be calculated non invasively from standard measurements. Fraction expired O₂ (FeO₂) and fraction inspired O₂ (FiO₂) and what other variable?**

Minute ventilation. $VO_2 = (FiO_2 - FeO_2)(VE)$.

❑❑ **Which energy substrate has the highest caloric density per gram?**

Fat.

❏❏ **The respiratory exchange ratio (RER) refers to the ratio of what two variables?**

VCO_2/VO_2.

❏❏ **The changes in RER are useful in determining what exercise phenomena?**

The anaerobic threshold.

❏❏ **List the advantages of using the cycle ergometer for exercise testing.**

Weight independent.
Less joint stress.
Less expensive.

❏❏ **Exercise testing is useful in Pediatrics. List four reasons to exercise a child.**

Reassurance that exercise is safe.
Evaluate surgical or medical therapies.
Investigate particular symptoms.
Probe for abnormalities specifically, heart, lung or muscle.

❏❏ **VE/VO_2 can add insight into the efficiency of the respiratory and muscular systems during exercise. In a pretest/ posttest on the same subject 12 weeks after aerobic training what changes would be seen in the VE/VO_2 during submaximal subanaerobic threshold exercise?**

The amount of VE needed for any given submaximal workload would be less.

❏❏ **Resistance training is useful for muscular hypertrophy. What are the three physiological adaptations that cause the increase in muscular size?**

Increase protein in the muscle fibers, increased capillaries and increased metabolic enzymes.

❏❏ **After three months of aerobic training, three days a week for thirty minutes a day at 75% of peak heart rate on a stress test, what change would you expect to see in maximum heart rate?**

There is no change in maximum heart rate.

❏❏ **What is the major regulatory enzyme for cellular glycolysis?**

Phosphofructokinase.

❏❏ **During human metabolism, high density (high caloric) energy is provided by what source?**

Triglycerides.

❐❐ **Describe the two major muscle types, including enzyme differences.**

Type I – slow twitch, high aerobic capacity because of increased enzyme lipoprotein lipase.
Type II – fast twitch, high glycolytic, increase phosphofructokinase.

❐❐ **During prolonged exercise (2 hours approximately 50 – 60 % of max VO_2), which fiber type would be doing a majority of the work?**

Slow twitch.

❐❐ **Describe simply the fuel utilization from the start of exercise to steady state exercise during mild exercise (40% - 50% VO_2 max).**

Muscle glycogen - Blood glucose - Free fatty acid.

❐❐ **Which neurohormones have an effect on heart rate during exercise?**

Catecholamines.

❐❐ **What major circulatory adjustment during exercise helps to increase the supply of blood for the exercising muscles?**

Shunting blood away from non essential areas, for example splanchnic circulation.

❐❐ **Define anatomical dead space.**

Airway passages of ambient air (nose, mouth and trachea) with no gas exchange potential.

❐❐ **Define physiological dead space.**

A portion of alveolar volume with poor ventilation to perfusion ratio.

❐❐ **T/F: Pulmonary circulation is a high pressure system, equal to systemic circulation.**

False. Pulmonary circulation is a low flow system, less than 25 mm Hg.

❐❐ **Define concentric muscular contractions.**

Where the muscle shortens with resistance.

❐❐ **Define eccentric muscular contractions.**

Where the muscle lengthens with resistance.

PROCEDURES

CASTING AND SPLINTING

❏❏ **T/F: Casts provide superior strength, durability and immobilization as compared to splints.**

True.

❏❏ **Identify some situations where the use of a splint or split cast may be indicated to allow for additional swelling.**

Fracture less than 48 hours old.
When additional soft tissue damage has occurred, e.g. crush injuries.
In patients who are unlikely to be able to comply with elevation.

❏❏ **T/F: Patients who have nondisplaced distal fibula fracture with significant swelling over the lateral malleolus should be casted immediately.**

False. When the swelling has resolved, there will be too much room in the cast. It is recommended to splint, elevate and then cast in 2-3 days.

❏❏ **T/F: If a cast is applied in order to maintain position in an unstable fracture, an x-ray should be taken after casting to ensure proper positioning.**

True.

❏❏ **When is the optimal time to check a cast?**

At 24 hours.

❏❏ **Describe components of the neurovascular examination that are essential before and after applying a cast.**

Check pulses.
Check capillary refill.
Check for light touch sensation.
Check for 2 point discrimination.

❏❏ **T/F: Cast padding is applied over a stockinette and can prevent ulceration over bony prominences and assist in avoiding burns when the cast is removed.**

True.

☐☐ **T/F: Since a stockinette is made of material that can breathe, it is not critical to have a smooth application against the skin.**

False. Any areas with wrinkles can cause indentation and ulceration in the skin.

☐☐ **T/F: In general, padding should be applied in a distal to proximal direction allowing for an overlapping of approximately one half width.**

True.

☐☐ **T/F: Fiberglass casts on the upper extremity need two layers for appropriate thickness, comfort and function.**

True.

☐☐ **T/F: Patients can have the injured extremity in a position of comfort and then be moved into a functional position after the cast tape has been applied.**

False. The functional position must be maintained as soon as the stockinette is applied to help avoid wrinkling and breakdown of the finished product.

☐☐ **T/F: To assist in maintaining position, hot water should be used with fiberglass casting material so that the material can set faster.**

False. Polymerization is an exothermic reaction. Warm to hot water can result in burns to the patient.

☐☐ **T/F: Casting materials should be rolled on from the distal end of the extremity to the proximal and overlap by one half width. Most casts need to be molded. This step is performed after the final roll has been applied.**

False. The molding must occur after the first roll is on to provide maximum comfort and to protect the skin from rubbing against the casting material.

☐☐ **T/F: When molding a cast one should use fingertip pressure to accurately provide the mold.**

False. Fingertip pressure can leave impressions or divots that lead to tissue necrosis. The palm of the hand is much better for this purpose.

☐☐ **T/F: When casting an extremity, there should be more stockinette than padding.**

True. Casting tape should be applied over the extremity only where cast padding has been applied. The stockinette can be rolled back over and incorporated into the cast to provide a well cushioned final product.

☐☐ **T/F: A cast care sheet should include advice to use of talcum powder to avoid itching.**

False. It should be reinforced that nothing should be placed in the cast.

❏❏ **T/F: Many patients, particularly children, are fearful that the cast saw will cut them. One can demonstrate that the cast saw does not rotate, but the sharp edges perform their task by vibrating.**

True.

❏❏ **T/F: The most common complication of cast removal is laceration requiring sutures.**

False. The most common complication is a burn. This may occur when either there is inadequate padding or the heat generated by the vibration of the cast saw is transmitted directly to the skin because of the use of too much pressure on the saw.

❏❏ **T/F: Patients can be instructed to press the involved extremity down towards a flat surface to provide more space when the contralateral side of the cast is being cut.**

True.

❏❏ **T/F: Once a cast is applied, it cannot be modified.**

False. A cast can be bivalved to allow for swelling, examination of lacerations and /or repadded for reuse after repeat x-rays are taken, particularly if non weight bearing indication is utilized.

❏❏ **Following an unwitnessed fall during a sporting event, a young athlete presents with a 1 week history of decreased use of his right hand. He is tender over the distal radius and x-ray studies confirm a torus fracture. What is the appropriate course of action?**

Apply a short arm cast.

❏❏ **In the above scenario, what is the correct position for wrist placement in the cast?**

Slight dorsiflexion.

❏❏ **T/F: The above cast should extend out to encompass the metacarpophalangeal joints.**

False. Only the radiocarpal joints need to be immobilized. Therefore this cast need only be anchored around the thumb.

❏❏ **T/F: The above cast should be molded into a perfect cylindrical shape.**

False. The cast should be elliptical to better accommodate the positions of the radius and ulna and to decrease the likelihood of pronation and supination that occur.

❏❏ **T/F: The casting of this injury should be from 3-6 weeks depending on the age of the patient and the injury.**

True.

❏❏ **A 21-year-old cyclist presents to you after falling on an outstretched hand. He has pain over the anatomic snuffbox. He cannot form a strong grip. Radiographic evaluation, including a navicular view reveal a scaphoid fracture. He tells you that this injury occurred at high speed. He does not have any swelling in the area and is a very compliant patient. What type of cast is appropriate?**

Long arm thumb spica cast.

❏❏ **T/F: In the above patient , the injured forearm and thumb should be placed in the neutral position as if he were gripping a pen.**

True. Thumb spicas do not need to have the thumb pointed upward.

❏❏ **T/F: In the above patient the wrist should be in functional position and the elbow at 90 degrees.**

True.

❏❏ **T/F: In the above patient the cast must extend from the left palmar crease to the mid biceps position.**

True.

❏❏ **T/F: After cutting a hole in the stockinette for the thumb, it is appropriate to apply a one inch stockinette or a 5/8 tubular gauze underneath the cast padding and extending halfway up the thumbnail. In doing so the nailbed of the thumb should be easily accessible to allow for assessment of capillary refill.**

True.

❏❏ **T/F: It is important to allow adequate space in the antecubital fossa when applying a long arm thumb spica in order to avoid impingement of the neurovascular bundle.**

True.

❏❏ **Two weeks after the application of a long arm thumb spica, this patient required reapplication. What physiologic change might account for this?**

Atrophy of the biceps.

❏❏ **T/F: Some authors suggests that if there is not high velocity involved with the original injury or after initial immobilization with a long arm thumb spica cast, that a short arm spica cast can be applied. In that case, the cast should be applied to the point just above the antecubital fossa.**

False. Short arm thumb spica casts are applied with two finger breadths space to allow for adequate flexion at the elbow without impingement.

❑❑ **T/F: The advantage of the long arm thumb spica is that it totally prevents pronation and supination from occurring at the wrist.**

True.

❑❑ **Despite adequate and immediate treatment with appropriate immobilization, avascular necrosis can occur in navicular fractures, even after 12 weeks of immobilization. If the x-ray still does not show adequate evidence of union at that time, the patient should be placed back in a long arm thumb spica cast for an additional 4 weeks.**

False. As with all fractures, patients should be counseled about likely outcomes. In cases of navicular fracture, even with appropriate treatment, there can be upwards of 40% incidence of nonunion. This will require referral to an orthopedic surgeon for probable surgery.

❑❑ **A 26-year-old athlete has been complaining of right lateral foot pain for a number of weeks. As a result he seeks consultation where you detect tenderness along the fifth metatarsal. X-ray studies do not identify a fracture site. One week later he took a misstep and with his foot in plantar flexion, he rolled over on the side of his foot. He returns to your facility with increased pain and now has swelling at the base of the fifth metatarsal. X ray at this time demonstrates a fracture approximately 1.5 cm from the styloid process of the fifth metatarsal. This is a true Jones fracture. He is not interested in consultation for a surgical approach, and since x ray does not demonstrate any sclerosis, he is an appropriate candidate for what type of casting?**

Short leg, non weight bearing cast

❑❑ **T/F: When applying stockinette for the above cast, one must place it from just past the toes up to the knee with the foot and ankle in neutral position with the knee flexed at 90 degrees with the slit across the front of the ankle to eliminate any folds or creases.**

True.

❑❑ **T/F: Cast padding should be applied starting at the distal end of the foot, straight across and overlapping by 50%.**

False. Since the foot is angled back from the great toe towards the fifth toe, and the metatarsal heads are further forward on the plantar aspect, the cast padding should be applied to accommodate these two factors.

❑❑ **T/F: The cast should be applied at least 2 fingerbreadths below the fibular head in order to avoid damage to the common peroneal nerve.**

True.

❑❑ **T/F: Extra padding is needed around the heel, malleoli, distal metatarsal heads and the proximal anterior tibia.**

True.

❑❑ **Identify important features of an appropriate mold for this cast.**

An arch around the medial aspect of the foot.
Around the Achilles tendon.
Around the heel.
Around the malleoli.
A triangular mold around the anterior tibia.

❑❑ **T/F: Since a period of up to 6 weeks of non weight bearing may be needed in this patient, the patient should be instructed in the correct use of crutches.**

True.

❑❑ **T/F: Muscle atrophy and the resulting fit of the cast may require reapplication of the cast during the 6 week period of immobilization.**

True.

❑❑ **If this same patient had also suffered an avulsion fracture of the fifth metatarsal and was in need of protection from further injury or if a nondisplaced distal fibula fracture was also present a short leg, weight bearing cast could be used. What would be the appropriate way to modify the already existing cast?**

Add reinforcement underneath the foot and heel to maintain the integrity of the cast.

❑❑ **To provide the modification referred to in the previous question, what steps would you take?**

Make reinforcement strips from the distal end of the cast to a point one inch up the back of the heel with 4-6 additional strips and incorporate them with the final roll.

❑❑ **T/F: When applying casting tape to the lower extremity, it should be applied so as not to add tension.**

False. Without a moderate degree of tension, the fiberglass will retract from the original application site, and there will be too much mobility in the cast.

❑❑ **T/F: When applying a short leg weight bearing cast, the ankle can be plantar flexed 10 degrees for comfort.**

False. This position will not allow for normal walking and will lead to shortening of the Achilles tendon and other post cast complications.

❏❏ **If the short leg cast is accidentally placed too tightly against the proximal fibula, what function will be affected?**

Eversion and dorsiflexion of the foot (foot drop).

❏❏ **T/F: Short leg casts can be used to treat Maisonneuve fractures.**

False. Maisonneuve fracture is a proximal fibular fracture along with bimalleolar fracture and potentially needs surgical intervention and / or long leg cast. Orthopedic consultation is recommended.

❏❏ **T/F: A short leg cast with the foot in equinus position is an acceptable alternative in a patient with a ruptured Achilles tendon, who is considered a poor surgical risk because of diabetes or severe peripheral vascular disease.**

True.

❏❏ **T/F: All short leg casts need only two layers of fiberglass because of it intrinsic strength.**

False. Lower extremity casts frequently need a third or fourth layer unless reinforcement layers are used as described above.

❏❏ **T/F: Patients should be instructed to leave the lower extremity in a dependent position to allow for better molding for the first twenty four hours after the cast has been applied.**

False. Elevation of the involved extremity is recommended to limit swelling.

❏❏ **A forty eight year old female runner complains of severe heel pain, made worse when she first gets up in the morning. She reports an " electrical " feeling from the heel to the arch of her foot. Physical examination confirms a diagnosis of plantar fasciitis. She refuses injection therapy and is unable to take nonsteroidals. She has used heel cups and stretches. Are there other options that may provide pain relief?**

Tension night splint.

❏❏ **T/F: When applying the above device, the knee should be fully extended.**

False. The knee needs to be flexed to allow maximum stretch of the gastroc since the medial lateral head originates on the lower portion of the femur.

❏❏ **Identify the features important to molding a tension night splint.**

Good arch support.
Molding around the Achilles tendon.
Extension of the device all the way out to the toes.

❑❑ **What modifications can be made to the tension night splint?**

1. Folding the fiberglass material to leave adequate room for the three toes on the lateral portion of the foot which do not need to be incorporated.
2. An adequate amount of spacing around the heel.
3. Maximum dorsiflexion at the ankle and the great toe.

❑❑ **What recommendations would you make to this patient regarding the use of the tension night splint?**

Apply splint at bedtime and remove when getting up in the morning.

❑❑ **An athlete has a severe inversion injury to the right ankle with significant swelling. There is tenderness over the lateral malleolus and you do not have x rays available but you do have splinting materials available. Identify some treatment options for this patient.**

Sugar tong splint.
Posterior splint.
Three way splint for initial immobilization.

❑❑ **What would be the advantage of choosing a sugar-tong splint in this patient?**

It reduces the amount of inversion and eversion.

❑❑ **What would be the advantage of a posterior splint in this patient?**

A posterior splint prevents too much plantar flexion.

❑❑ **What would be the advantage of a three way splint for initial immobilization in this patient?**

The benefit of a 3-way immobilization system is that with use of adequate padding around the malleoli you can reduce the amount of swelling, maintain the ankle at 90 degrees as well as prevent inversion or eversion until further evaluation can be performed.

PROCEDURES

JOINT ASPIRATION AND INTRAARTICULAR INJECTION

❏❏ **Identify indications for joint aspiration.**

To evaluate synovial fluid and differentiate the cause of joint effusion.
To remove exudative fluid form a septic joint.
To relieve pain in a grossly swollen joint.

❏❏ **T/F: If multiple joints are inflamed, the elbow is generally the easiest to aspirate.**

False. The knee is generally considered to be the easiest to aspirate.

❏❏ **T/F: Evaluation of joint fluid can generally differentiate between rheumatic, infectious, traumatic and crystal induced causes of effusion.**

True.

❏❏ **T/F: While the metacarpophalangeal (MCP) joints can be aspirated , the smaller proximal interphalangeal (PIP) and distal interphalangeal (DIP) joints are not amenable to aspiration.**

False. While it often requires a more experienced clinician, all of the joints of the digits and even the sternoclavicular joint can be tapped for diagnostic evaluation.

❏❏ **What is the upper frequency limit that is considered safe for injecting corticosteroids into a weight bearing joint?**

There is no absolute consensus on how many injections are safe, however many use 3 times a year as the upper limit.

❏❏ **T/F: Repeated injections of corticosteroids into a joint can cause osteoporosis and cartilage damage.**

True.

❏❏ **Identify contraindication to injection of corticosteroids into weight bearing joints.**

Cellulitis of the overlying soft tissue.
Bacteremia.
Anticoagulant therapy.

☐☐ **What structures are at risk of injury during joint aspiration or injection?**

Veins and arteries.
Nerves.
Articular cartilage.

☐☐ **T/F: Intraarticular injections typically consist of Xylocaine or Marcaine, a corticosteroid and epinephrine.**

False. Epinephrine is not used for intra-articular injections.

☐☐ **T/F: The long tendon of the biceps is injected just below the coracoid process and the short tendon of the biceps is injected in the bicipital groove.**

False.

☐☐ **T/F: Despite its name, the subacromial bursa of the shoulder is actually found just superior to the acromion process when aspirating or injecting for bursitis.**

False. It is found inferior to the acromion.

☐☐ **When injecting steroid anesthetic for carpal tunnel syndrome, you know you are in the correct location when the patient feels pain in the palm or fingertips.**

False. The needle should be withdrawn and repositioned, as the median nerve should not be injected but rather the carpal tunnel.

☐☐ **T/F: The elbow is usually easier to inject when it is flexed.**

True.

☐☐ **When the knee is flexed at 90 degrees, what is the best site for aspiration and injection?**

Superior to the tibial plateau and medial to the infrapatellar tendon.

☐☐ **With the knee fully extended, what is the usual site used for aspiration?**

On the medial aspect of the knee at a point halfway between the mid patella and the underlying femoral condyle.

☐☐ **Where is the preferred site for aspiration of the ankle?**

Injection is performed between the medial malleolus and the extensor hallucis tendon with the needle aimed downward and laterally.

❏❏ **T/F: The glenohumeral joint of the shoulder should only be aspirated from an anterior approach.**

False. The joint can be entered anteriorly with the shoulder rotated externally and the needle directed medial to the humerus and inferior to the tip of the coracoid. Using a posterior approach, the needle is inserted 4 cm medial to the lateral aspect of the shoulder and 1 cm below the posterior aspect of the acromion.

❏❏ **Identify three important landmarks for injecting the wrist using a posterior approach.**

Distal border of the radius.
Distal border of the ulna.
Extensor pollicis longus tendon.

❏❏ **T/F: It is not advisable to inject corticosteroids into an unstable joint nor into one that has marked juxta-articular osteoporosis.**

True.

❏❏ **Identify some potential sequelae following intra-articular injections of corticosteroids.**

Charcot like ("steroid") arthropathy.
Tendon rupture.
Fat Necrosis.

❏❏ **Tenosynovitis (trigger finger) responds best to surgery, followed by local injection with methylprednisolone and triamcinolone. What are the relative response rates?**

Injection 70 - 80 %.
Surgery 90%.

❏❏ **Describe the proper technique for injection of tenosynovitis.**

1. Sterile preparation with Betadine scrub followed by use of an alcohol wipe.
2. Injection at the A-1 pulley in the palm over the metacarpal head through the flexor tendon.
3. Confirmation of placement with passive flexion of the appropriate finger to elicit movement of the needle.
4. Injection of anesthetic followed by steroid just above the flexor tendon.

❏❏ **What is the most common adverse reaction to injection of tenosynovitis?**

Pain at the injection site.

❏❏ **T/F: After a diagnosis of gout or pseudogout has been made by evaluation of joint fluid, it is never necessary to aspirate or inject that patients joints again.**

False. Even though oral therapy is the treatment of choice, therapeutic aspiration of an acutely inflamed joint may provide instant pain relief, and some patients who cannot tolerate oral therapy may be helped by local steroid injection.

❏❏ **What type of crystal is most difficult to identify in aspirated fluid from an inflamed joint?**

Calcium hydroxyapatite.

❏❏ **A 17-year-old, sexually active male athlete presents with an acutely inflamed left knee with an obvious effusion. Gram stain of the synovial fluid fails to show any organisms. What is the most appropriate course of action?**

Start empiric ceftriaxone IV once a day and await culture results. In this patient N. gonorrhea is the most likely organism. Gram stain and culture of the joint aspirate may be negative. A blood culture should also be done.

❏❏ **A 27-year-old athlete presents with wrist pain. Finkelstein's sign is positive on exam. Part of the treatment regimen includes injection of methylprednisolone. What site would you choose for the injection?**

This patient has de Quervain's tenosynovitis, not carpal tunnel syndrome. Therefore the injection should be given into the tendon sheath of the abductor pollicis longus and extensor pollicus brevis tendons.

❏❏ **An adult baseball player presents with anterior shoulder pain that radiates into the lateral upper arm muscles. Injection of methylprednisolone under the anterolateral aspect of the acromion relieves the pain. What is the most likely diagnosis?**

Subdeltoid bursitis.

❏❏ **A 45-year-old obese female patient presents to your office with a long history of nonspecific knee pain that has been much worse for the past three days. Point tenderness is present along the distal medial plateau and it is relieved by local injection. What is the most likely diagnosis?**

Anserine bursitis.

❏❏ **What is the most likely organism to be identified in the joint aspirate from a 23 year old male athlete with reactive arthritis, urethritis and conjunctivitis (Reiter's syndrome)?**

Chlamydia trachomatis.

❏❏ **What is the most likely organism to be identified in the joint aspirate of a 15-year-old, sexually active female athlete with septic arthritis of the shoulder?**

Neisseria gonorrheae.

PROTECTIVE AND SUPPORTIVE EQUIPMENT

❏❏ **Name the important factors in choosing protective sports equipment.**

Cleanliness.
Fit.
Use.
Condition.

❏❏ **Who is responsible for safety when an athlete provides his/her own equipment?**

Certified athletic trainer.

❏❏ **What is the purpose of sports protective equipment?**

Protection from injury and reinjury.

❏❏ **Identify important design factors.**

Increased impact area.
Transferred of dispersed impact area.
Limitation of relative motion of a body part.
Absorbance of energy.
Resist absorption of viruses, fungi and bacteria.
Reduce friction between surfaces.

❏❏ **What determines equipment efficacy?**

Thickness.
Density.
Temperature energy absorbance.

❏❏ **How does the nature of the sport influence your choice of materials?**

Soft, low density materials provide comfort and are appropriate for low impact forces. Firmer density materials are appropriate for high impact forces, but are less cushioning and comfortable. Highly resilient materials are appropriate for repeated trauma.

❏❏ **What material is best suited for shock absorbance?**

Closed cell foam.

❑❑ **What is the purpose of layering?**

Layering, while expensive and requiring extensive maintenance, provides maximal shock absorption.

❑❑ **What materials are best suited for body part splinting?**

Fiberglass or plaster.

❑❑ **What problems can occur from their extended use?**

Dermatitis, blisters, infections, maceration, ulceration, abrasions.

❑❑ **What organizations have specific rules governing the use of hard and soft materials for body protection?**

National Collegiate Athlete Association.
National Federation of State High School Association.
United States Olympic Committee.
National Association of Intercollegiate Athletes.

❑❑ **Who is responsible for the enforcement of the regulations at a competition?**

On site referee.

❑❑ **What organization sets the standards for baseball, softball, football and lacrosse helmets?**

National Operating Committee on standards for Athletic Equipment.

❑❑ **Which sports require the use of helmets?**

Amateur boxing, martial arts, bicycling, white water sports, softball, baseball, men's lacrosse and football.

❑❑ **T/F: The single bar football helmet meets minimum protection standards.**

False.

❑❑ **Name some of the criteria for correctly fitting a football helmet.**

Hair should be cut and wet.
Inflate air bladder.
Select proper sized shell and adjust appropriately.
Ensure snug fit.

❑❑ **When is a helmet fitted appropriately?**

Firm resistance should be felt when the helmet is moved side to side and when a tongue depressor is inserted between the pads and the face.

❏❏ **What organizations monitor ice hockey helmet standards?**

American Society for Testing Material.
Hockey Equipment Certification Council.

❏❏ **What sports require protective eye wear?**

No interscholastic or intercollegiate sport require eyewear although it is recommended for all racquet sports, basketball, soccer, baseball, soccer, cycling, martial arts and athletes with monocular vision or vision in only one eye.

❏❏ **What organism is associated with aquatics and use of contact lenses?**

Acanthamoeba.

❏❏ **Which sports require ear protection?**

Wrestling, martial arts, boxing, water polo and target/ skeet shooting.

❏❏ **What sports require the use of an intra-oral mouthguard?**

All interscholastic and intercollegiate football, ice hockey, men's and women's lacrosse and field hockey.

❏❏ **What types of intra-oral mouthguard are available?**

Pressure formed laminated type which is most effective and expensive requiring special training; vacuum-formed which are less expensive and easier to design but over time lose their elastic memory.

❏❏ **Which sports require throat and neck protectors?**

The NCAA requires softball and baseball catchers to wear built-in or attachable throat guards on their masks.

❏❏ **What is the most critical equipment factor in preventing brachial plexus injuries?**

Properly fitted shoulder pads is the most critical factor followed by a cervical neck roll and collar.

❏❏ **What type of shoulder pads are recommended for quarterbacks and receivers?**

Lightweight flat shoulder pads are appropriate for quarterbacks and receivers.

❏❏ **What type of shoulder pads are appropriate for linemen?**

Cantilever pads are appropriate for linemen.

❏❏ **What are the requirements for elbow protection at the high school and college level?**

No rigid material can be worn at the elbow or below unless covered on all sides by closed - cell foam padding.

❏❏ **Are sports bras effective in preventing sore, tender breasts post exercise?**

No, despite the prevention of excessive vertical and horizontal breast motion during exercise.

❏❏ **What is an important side effect of inappropriately placed thigh pads?**

Genital injury due to the placement of the asymmetrical portion of the medial aspect.

❏❏ **What are the functional categories of knee braces?**

Rehabilitative (RKB), prophylactic (PKB), and functional (FKB).

❏❏ **Describe some of the indications for RKB, PKB and FKBs?**

1. RKBs provide absolute immobilization at a selected angle after surgery, permit controlled range of motion through predetermined arcs and prevent accidental loading in non weight bearing patients.
2. PKBs protect the medial collateral ligament.
3. FKBs are used widely to protect moderate ACL injuries and post surgical ACL repair/reconstruction cases.

❏❏ **Is the routine use of PKBs effective?**

The AAOS has concluded that the routine use of PKBs has not proven effective in reducing either the number or severity of knee injuries and may in some instances be a contributing factor to injury.

❏❏ **What is the clinical use of patellar braces?**

Relief of anterior knee pain syndrome.

❏❏ **Distinguish semi-rigid ankle orthosis from lace-up braces?**

The semi-rigid orthosis limits inversion and eversion whereas the lace-up brace limits all ankle motion.

❏❏ **What is the durability of surgical ankle strapping?**

The maximal tensile strength of ankle strapping is lost after 20 minutes or more of exercise.

❑❑ **What are the key factors in athletic footwear selection?**

Wear socks typically worn in competition.
Fit shoes at the end of workout or end of day.
Widest shoepart should coincide with widest footpart.
Eyelets should be spaced at least 1 inch apart with normal lacing.
Pick a moderately supportive sole.
The heel counter should be made of thermoplastic material.
Allow 2 - 3 days of walking for foot adaptation to occur.

❑❑ **How often should athletic shoes be replaced by runners?**

Every 3 months or 500 miles for avid runners; every 6 months for recreational runners.

❑❑ **What type of shoewear is appropriate for an overpronator?**

Greater medial side control.

❑❑ **What shoewear is recommended for a flexible low arch?**

Straight last, very firm midsole and strong hindfoot stability.

BIBLIOGRAPHY

The Team Physician

Team Physician Consensus Statement. American Academy of Family Physicians, American Academy of Orthopedic Surgeons, American College of Sports Medicine, American Orthopedic Society of Sports Medicine and American Osteopathic Society of Sports Medicine 2000

Certified Athletic Trainers in Secondary Schools, Report 5 of the Council on Scientific Affairs (A-98). AMA 2000

Birrer, R.B. (ED) 2nd edition, Sports Medicine for the Primary care Physician, Boca Raton, Fla: CRC, 1994

Exercise Physiology, Anatomy & Biomechanics, Growth & Development

American Academy of Orthopaedic Surgeons Athletic Training & Sports Medicine, 2nd edition, Rosemont, Illinois 1991

Garrett, WE, Jr. and Kirkendall, DT, eds, Exercise and Sports Science, Lippincott, Williams & Wilkins, Philadelphia, Pennsylvania 2000

Garrick, JG and Webb, DR, Sports Injuries – Diagnosis & Management, W.B. Saunders Co., Philadelphia 1999

Grant, JCB, Grant's Atlas of Anatomy, 5th edition, Williams & Wilkins, Baltimore, 1962

Greene, WB, ed, Essentials of Musculoskeletal Care – 2nd edition., American Academy of Orthopedic Surgeons, Rosemont, Illinois 2001

Kendall, FP, McCreary, EK and Provance, PG, Muscle Testing & Function, 4th edition, Williams & Wilkins, Baltimore, Maryland 1993

Kibler, WB, The Sport Preparticipation Fitness Examination, Human Kinetics Books, Champaign, Illinois 1990

Malina, RM and Bouchard, C, Growth, Maturation and Physical Activity, Human Kinetics Books, Champaign, Illinois 1991

McArdle, WD, Katch FI, and Katch, VL, Essentials of Exercise Physiology, 2nd edition, Lippincott, Williams & Wilkins, Baltimore 2000

McArdle, WD, Katch, FL, Katch VL, Sports Exercise & Nutrition, Lippincott, Williams & Wilkins, Philadelphia 1999

Mellion, MB, Office Management of Sports Injuries & Athletic Problems, Hanley & Belfus, Inc, Philadelphia, PA 1988

Mellion, M, Walsh, WM, Shelton, GL, The Team Physician's Handbook, 2nd edition, Hanley & Belfus, Philadelphia 1997

Mellion, MB, Sports Medicine Secrets, 2nd edition, Hanley & Belfus, Philadelphia 1999

Report of the Ross Symposium. Muscle Development: Nutritional Alternatives to Anabolic Steroids; Ross Laboratories, Columbus, Ohio 1988

Strohmeyer HS, Williams K and Schaub-George D. Developmental sequences for catching a small ball : a prelongitudinal study. *Research Quarterly for Exercise and Sport.* 62(3):257-266, 1991

Sullivan, J.A. and Anderson, SJ,(eds), Care of the Young Athlete, American Academy of Orthopedic Surgeons and American Academy of Pediatrics, Illinois 2000

Teitz, CC, Ed, Scientific Foundations of Sports Medicine, BC Decker, Philadelphia, PA 1989

Pharmacotherapeutics

Care of the Young Athlete. American Academy of Pediatrics. American Academy of Orthopedic Surgeons 2000

Henderson, H, Therapeutic Drugs, Clinics in Sports Medicine, 1998; 17 (2): 229 – 243

Ergogenic Agents

Athletic Drug Reference. Glaxo Wellcome, Clean Data Publishers, Inc 1999

Bhasin, S, Storer, T, Berman, N, Callegari, C, Clevanger B, Phillips, J, Bunnell, T, Tricker, R, Shirazi, A, Casaburi, R, The Effects of supraphysiologic doses of testosterone on muscle size and strength in normal men., NEJM 1996; 335 (1): 1-8

Headley, S, Massad, S, Nutritional supplements for athletes. National Association for Sports & Physical Education 1999

Juhn, M, Tarnopolsky, M, Oral creatine supplementation and athletic performance: A critical review. Clin J Sports Med 1998; 8: 286-297

Juhn, M, Tarnopolsky,M, Potential side effects of oral creatine supplementation: A critical review., Clin J Sports Med 1998;8: 298-304

Kernan, W, Viscoli, C, Brass, L, Broderick, J, Brott, T, Feldman, E, Morgenstern L, Wilterdink, J, Horowitz, R, Phenylpropanolamine and the risk of hemorrhagic stroke, NEJM 2000; 343(25): 1826-1832

Laseter, J, Russell, J,Anabolic steroid induced tendon pathology: a review of the literature, Med Sci Sports Exer 1991; 23 (1): 1-3

Leder, B, Longoscope, C, Catlin, D, Ahrens, B, Schoenfeld, D, Finkelstein, J, Oral androstenedione administration and serum testosterone concentrations in young men. JAMA2000; 283 (6): 779- 782

Mochizuki, R, Richter, K, Cardiomyopathy and cerebrovascular accident associated with anabolic-androgenic steroid use. Phys and Sports med 1988; 16 (11): 109-114

Melchert, R, Herron, T, Welder, A, The effect of anabolic-androgenic steroids on primary myocardial cell cultures. Med Sci Sports Exer 1992; 24 (2): 206-212

Office of the Director, National Institutes of Health. Dietary supplements for Physically Active People. US Government Printing. June 1996

Rogol, A., Yesalis, C., Anabolic-androgenic steroids and the adolescent, Ped Annals 1992; 21(3): 175-188

Terjung, R,(chairman), American College of Sports Medicine Roundtable. The Physiological and Health Effects of Oral Creatine Supplementation, Med Sci Sports Exer 2000; 32 (3): 706-717

USOC Guide to Prohibited Substances. United States Olympic Committee 2000

Walker, L, Bemben, M, Bemben, D, Knehans, A, Chromium picolinate effects on body composition and muscular performance in wrestlers, Med Sci Sports Exer 1998; 30(12): 1730-1737

Conditioning & Training

American Academy of Pediatrics, Athletic Participation by Children and Adolescents who have systemic hypertension, Pediatrics 1997; 4:637-638

American Academy of Pediatrics, Medical Conditions affecting Sports Participation, Pediatrics 1994; 5: 757-760

Baechle, T, Essentials of Strength Training and Conditioning. National Strength & Conditioning Association, Human Kinetics 1994

Care of the Young Athlete, American Academy of Pediatrics. American Academy of Orthopedic Surgeons 2000

Evans, C, Karunaratne, H, Exercise stress testing for the family physician: Part I, Performing the Test, Am Fam Phys 1992; 1:121-132

Evans, C, Karunaratne, H, Exercise stress testing for the family physician: Part II, Interpretation of the results. Amer Fam Phys 1992; 2: 679-688

Fisher, A, Jensen, C, Scientific basis of Athletic conditioning, Lea & Febiger 1990

Fitts, R, Widrick, J, Muscle Mechanics : Adaptations with Exercise Training, Exercise & Sports Science Reviews 1996: 24; 427-474

Hagberg, J et al, Effect of Weight Training on Blood Pressure and Hemodynamics in Hypertensive Adolescents, J Peds 1984; 104: 147-151

Kramer, W et al, Strength and Power Training: Physiological mechanisms of adaptation, Exercise and Sports Science Reviews 1996: 24; 363 -397

McArdle, W, Exercise Physiology 3rd edition, Lea & Febiger 1991

North, T, et al, Effects of Exercise on Depression, Exercise and Sports Science reviews 1990:18; 379-415

Orenstein, D, Exercise Conditioning in Children with Asthma, J Peds 1985; 106:556-558

Sjodin, B, Onset of blood lactate accumulation and marathon running performance, Int J Sports Med 1981; 2:23-26

Sleamaker, R, Serious training for Serious Athletes, Human Kinetics 1989

Tip[ton, C, Exercise, Training and Hypertension: an update, Exer Sports Sci Rev 1991;19: 447-505

Trueth, M et al, Effects of Training on Intra-abdominal adipose tissue in obese prepubertal girls. Med Sci Sports Exer 1998: 1738-1732

Van Etten, L, et al, Effect of Body Build on Weight Training induced adaptations in body composition and muscular strength, Med Sci Sports Exer. 1994: 515-520

Wolfe, R, Anaerobic Threshold as a predictor of athletic performance in prepubertal female runners, AJDC 1986;140:922-924

Nutrition

Heimburger, DC, Weinsier, RL, Handbook of Clinical Nutrition, 3rd edition, Mosby, N.Y. 1997

Mc Ardle, WD, Katch, FI, Katch, VL, Sports and Exercise Nutrition, Lippincott, Willians and Wilkins, Philadelphia, PA 1999

Williams, SR, Nutrition and Diet Therapy – 8th edition, Mosby, N.Y.1997

Exercise Prescriptions

American College of Sports Medicine (Position Statement). The recommended quantity and quality of exercise for developing and maintaining cardiorespiratory and muscular fitness and flexibility in healthy adults, Med Sci Sports Exerc 1998; 30 (6): 975 – 991

American College of Sports Medicine (Position Stand): Exercise and Type II diabetes, Med Sci Sport Exerc, 2000; 32(6): 1345-1360

American College of Sports Medicine (Position Stand): Exercise for patients with coronary artery disease, Med Sci Sport Exerc 1994;26(3): I-V

Franklin, BA, Whaley, MH, Howley ET, (eds), ACSM's Guidelines for Exercise Testing and Prescription 6th edition, Lippincott, Williams & Wilkins 2000

Fu,FH, Stone, DA, (ed) Sports Injuries, Williams and Wilkins 1994

Hertzer, NR, Beven, EG, Young, JR, Coronary artery disease in peripheral vascular patients: a classification of 1000 coronary angiograms and results of surgical management., Ann Surg 199:223-233 1984

Pate, RR, et al, Physical Activity and Public Health. A Recommendation From the Centers for Disease Control and Prevention and the American College of Sports Medicine, JAMA 1995; 273(5): 402-407

Physical Activity and Cardiovascular Health. NIH Consensus Statement 1995 Dec 18 - 20; 13(3): 1-33

Sallis, RE, Massimino, F, (ed), ACSM's Essentials of Sports Medicine, Mosby 1997

Epidemiology

Backx, FJG, Epidemiology of paediatric sports related injuries , IN: Bar-Or, O (ed), The Child and Adolescent Athlete, Blackwell Science 1996

Bak, K, Nontraumatic glenohumeral instability and coracoacromial impingement in swimmers, Scand J Med Sci Sports, 6: 13 1996

Beunen, G, Malina, R.M., Growth and physical performance relative to the timing of the adolescent spurt, Exer Sport Sci Rev 16: 503 1998

Burgess – Milliron, MJ, MurphySB., Biomechanical considerations of youth sports injuries, IN; Bar Or, O (ed), The Child and Adolescent Athlete, Blackwell Science, 1996

Cahill, B.R., Osteolysis of the distal part of the clavicle in male athletes, J Bone Joint Surg Am 64A: 1053, 1982

Carson, WG, Gasser, SI, Little leaguer's shoulder: A report of 23 cases, Am J Sports Med 26: 575 1998

Di Fiori, JP, Overuse injuries in Children and Adolescents. Phys Sportsmed 27: 75-89, 1999

Micheli, LJ, Fehlandt, AF, Overuse injuries to tendons and apophyses in children and adolescents. Clin Sports Med 11: 713, 1992

Patel, DR, Greydanus, DE, The adolescent athlete, IN: Hoffmann, AD, Greydanus, DE (eds), Adolescent Medicine, Stamford, CT, Appleton – Lange 1997

Smith, JA, Hu, SS, Management of spondylolysis and spondylolisthesis in the pediatric and adolescent population, Ortho Clin North Am 30: 487, 1999

Event Administration & Injury Prevention

Arendt, EA, Stress fractures and the female athlete, Clin Orthop, 2000 Mar (372): 131-8

ASDA Newsletter v 312 – listing punishments for drug offenses

Kannus, P, Etiology and Pathophysiology of Chronic Tendon Disorders in Sports, Scand J. Med Sci Sports 1997;7: 78-85

Livingston, S, Pauli, LL, Pruce, I, Epilepsy and Drowning in Children, Br Med J , 1977; 2: 515-516

Sullivan, JA, Anderson SJ,(ed), Care of the Young Athlete, American Academy of Orthopaedic Surgeons. American Academy of Pediatrics

Zeni, AI, Street, CC, Dempsey, RL, Staton, M, Stress Injury to the Bone among Women Athletes, Phys Med Rehab Clin N. Am, 2000 Nov; 11 (4): 929-47

Triage and On Field Emergencies

Abrunzo, TJ, Commotio cordis: The single most common cause of traumatic death in youth baseball, Am J Dis Child 1991; 145: 1279-1282

Anderson, MK, Hall, SJ, Fundamentals of Sports Injury Management, Williams & Wilkins, Phil 1997

Bishop PJ, Wells, RP., Cervical Spine fractures: mechanisms, neck loads and methods of prevention, IN: Castaldi, CR, Hoerner, EF (ed) Safety in Ice Hockey, ASTM, Philadelphia 1989: 71-83

Bracken, MB, Shepard, MJ, Collins, WF et al, A randomized controlled trial of methylprednisolone or naloxone in the treatment of acute spinal cord injury. Results of the Second National Acute Spinal Cord Injury Study, NEJM 1990; 322:1405-1411

Committee on Trauma, American College of Surgeons. Advanced Trauma Life Support Manual, American College of Surgeons, CHicage, 1996: 1-243

Cooper, DE, Warren, RF, Barnes, R, traumatic subluxation of the hip resulting in aseptic necrosis and condrylolysis in a professional football player, Am J Sports Med 1991; 19: 322-324

Gerberich, SG, Priest, JD, Boen, JR et al, Concussion incidences and severity in secondary school varsity football players, Am J Public Health 1993; 73: 1370-1375

Green, ED, Simson, LR, Lkellerman, HH, et al, Cardiac concussion following softball blow to the chest, Ann Emerg Med 1990;9: 155-157

Karofsky, PS, Death of a high school hockey player, Phys Sportmed 1990; 18: 99-103

Larson,RL, Dislocations and ligamentous injuries to the knee, IN: Rockwood,, CA, Green, DP (eds), Fractures, JB Lippincott, Philadelphia 1995: 1182

Mandelbaum, BR, Wrist pain in the gymnast, Am J Sports Med 1989; 17(3):305-317

Marion, DW, Darby, J, Yonas, H, Acute regional cerebral blood flow changes caused by severe head injuries, J Neurosurg 1991; 74: 406-414

Nagobads, VG, Head Injuries and protective face masks for goalies in ice hockey, Presented IIHF Medical Congress, Fribourge, Switzerland, April 21, 1990

Rimel, RN, Giordani, B, Barth, JT et al, Disability caused by minor head injury, Neurosurgery 1991;9:221-228

Sallis, RE, Massimino, F, ACSM's Essentials of Sports Medicine, Mosby, NY 1997

Stenger, A, Bo's hip dislocates stellar athletic career, Phys Sportmed 1991;19(5): 17-18

Stewart, WJ, Aseptic necrosis of the head of the femur following traumatic dislocation of the hip joint case reported in experimental studies. J Bone Surg 1933; 15: 413-438

Tator, CH, Edmonds, VE, Lapczak, L, Tator, IB, Spinal injuries in ice hockey players 1966-1987, 1990

Acute Musculoskeletal Injuries

Mellion, MB, Walsh, WM, Shelton, GL, The Team Physician's Handbook, Hanley & Belfus, Inc. 1997

Nelson, C, Which athletes are most at risk for stress fractures?, Sports Medicine Digest, 2001, Vol 23 (1): 1-5

Netter, FH, The CIBA Collection of Medical Illustrations Vol 8, Musculoskeletal System Part 1

Reid, DC, Sports Injury, Assessment and Rehabilitation, Churchhill Livingstone Inc., 1992

Sallis, RE, Massimino, F, ACSM's Essentials of Sports Medicine,Mosby – Year Book Inc, 1997

Schoene, ML, Nelson, C, High levels of osteoarthritis among female soccer players following an ACL tear, Sports Medicine Digest 2000, Vol 22 (12): 133-138

Sullivan, JA, Anderson, SJ, Care of the Young Athlete, The American Academy of Pediatrics and the American Academy of Orthopedic Surgeons 2000: 309-321; 338-339; 349-364

Tator, CH,et al, Hockey injuries of the spine in Canada ,Canadian Medical Association Journal 2000; 162: 787-8

Chronic Medical Problems

American Diabetes Association. Clinical Practice Recommendations 2001, Diabetes care 2001; 24 (Suppl 1): S5- S133

Fields, KB, Fricker, PA, Medical Problems in Athletes, Blackwell Science, Malden MA 1997

Johnson, R, Sports Medicine in Primary Care, WB Saunders Co, Philadelphia 2000

Marolf, GA, Kuhn, A, White, RD, Exercise Testing in Special Populations: Athletes, women and the elderly, Primary Care 28;2001: 55-72

Mellion, MB, Walsh, WM, Shelton, GL, The Team Physician's Handbook, 2nd edition, Hanley & Belfus, Inc, Phil 1997

Smith, DM, Kovan, JR, Rich, BSE, Tanner, SM, Preparticipation Physican Evaluation, 2nd edition, McGraw Hill Companies, Minneapolis 1997

White, RD, Evans, CH, Performing the exercise test, Primary Care 28; 2001:29-53

Williams, RA, The Athlete and Heart Disease – Diagnosis, Evaluation & Management, Lippincott, Williams & Wilkins, Philadelphia 1999

Preparticipation Physical Examination

American Academy of Pediatrics Committee on Sports Medicine and Fitness: Medical conditions affecting sports participation, Pediatrics 1994; 94(5): 757-760

American Medical Society for Sports Medicine, American Orthopedic Society for Sports Medicine: Human immunodeficiency virus and other blood borne pathogens in sports. Clin J Sports Med 1995: 5(3): 199-204

Arendt, E, Dick, R, Knee injury patterns among men and women in collegiate basketball and soccer. Am J Sports Med 1995; 23: 694-701

Brent,BS, Sudden death screening, Med Clin North America 1994: 78(2): 267-288

26th Bethesda Conference: Recommendations for Determining eligibility for competition in athletes with cardiovascular abnormalities. January 6-7, 1994, Med Sci Sports Exer 1994; 26 (10 Suppl): S 223-283

Corrado, D, Basso, C, Schiavon, M, Theine, G, Screening for hypertrophic cardiomyopathy in young athletes, NEJM 1998; 339(6): 364-369

Eichner, E.R., Sickle cell trait, exercise and altitude, Phys Sportsmed 1986; 14 (11): 144-157

Ferenchick, GS, Adelman, S, Myocardial infarction associated with anabolic steroid use in a previously healthly 37 year old weight lifter, Am Heart J 1992; 124 (2): 507-508

Goldberg, B, Saranti, A, Witman, P, et al, Preparticipation sports assessment: An objective evaluation. Pediatrics 1980; 66 (5) 736-745

Gomez, JE, Landry, GL, Bernhardt, DT, Critical evaluation of the 2 minute orthopedic screening examination, Am J Dis Child 1993; 147(10): 1109-1113

Guidelines for the Prevention of Transmission of human immunodeficiency virus and Hepatitis B virus to healthcare and public safety workers, Morb Mortal Wkly Rep 1989; 38 (supp 6): 1-37

Hara, JH, Puffer, JC, The Preparticipation physical examination, In: Mellion, MB, ed, Office Management of Sports Injuries and Athletic Problems. Philadelphia, Hanley & Belfus 1988

Hein, K., Commentary on adolescent acquired immune deficiency syndrome: The next wave of the human immunodeficiency virus epidemic ? J Pediatr 1989; 114: 144

Kelly, JP, Nichols, JS, Filley, CM, et al, Concussion in sports: guidelines for the prevention of catastrophic outcome, JAMA 1991; 266 (20): 2867-2869

Kiser, C, Shank, M, Kraemer, W, et al, Effects of chewing tobacco on heart rate and blood pressure during exercise, J Sports Med Phys Fitness 1986; 26: 384-396

Krochuck DP, The preparticipation athletic examination: a closer look, Pediatr Ann 1997: 26(4) 37-49

Maron, BJ, Casey, SA, Poliac, LC, Gohman, TE, Alquist, AK, Aeppli, EM, Clinical course of hypertrophic cardiomyopathy in a regional United States cohort, JAMA 1999; 281 (7): 650-655

Maron, BJ, Thompson, PD, Puffer, JC, McGrew, CA, Strong, WB, Douglas, PS, et al, Cardiovascular preparticipation screening of competitive athletes. A statement for health professionals from the Sudden Death Committee and Congenital Cardiac Defects Committee, American Heart Association. Circulation 1996; 94: 850 -6
Addendum appears in Circulation 1998; 97:2294

McCormick, DP, Ivey, FM, Gold, DM et al, The Preparticipation sports examination in Special Olympic athletes, Texas Med 1988; 84 (4): 39-43

Mc Keag, DB ,Preseason physical examination for the prevention of Sports Injuries, Sports Med 1985; 2(6): 413-431

Mittenburg, W, Burton, DB, A survey of treatment for post concussion syndrome. Brain Injury 1994; 8(5): 429 -437

National Center for Health Statistics. Vital Statistics of the United States 1989, Vol II: Mortality, Part A. Washington D.C., Public Health Service 1993

National Collegiate Athletic Association: 1998-1999 Sports Medicine Handbook. Overland Park, KS, National Collegiate Athletic Association 1998

Rupp, NT, Brudno, DS, Guill, MF, The Value of Screening for Risk of Exercise induced Asthma in High School Athletes, Ann Allergy 1993; 70 (4): 339-342

Sallis, RE, Jones,K, Knopp, W, Burners: Offensive strategy for an underreported injury, Phys Sportsmed 1992; 20(11): 47 -55

Smith, DM, Kovan, JR, Rich, BSE, Tanner, SM, Preparticipation Physical Evaluation Monograph, Ed2. Minneapolis, MN, American Academy of Family Physicians, American Academy of Pediatrics, American Medical Society for Sports Medicine, American Orthopedic Society for Sports Medicine, American Osteopathic Academy of Sports Medicine 1997

Smith, J, Laskowski, E, The Preparticipation physical examination: Mayo Clinic experience with 2739 examinations, Mayo Clinic Proceedings 1998; 72:419-429

Squire, DL, Eating disorders, In: Mellion, MB , ed, Sports Medicine Secrets, Philadelphia, Hanley & Belfus, Inc; St Louis, Mosby 1993; 136 – 141

Stevens, MB, Smith, GN, The Preparticipation sports assessment, Fam Pract Recert 1986; 8(3): 63-88

Tanji, JL, The preparticipation exam: special concerns for the Special Olympics, Phys Sportsmed 1991; 19 (7): 61-68

Torg, JS, Management Guidelines for Athletic Injuries to the Cervical spine, Clin Sports med 1987;6(1): 53-60

Van Camp, SP, Bloor, CM, Mueller, FO, Cantu, RC, Olson, HG, Nontraumatic sports deaths in high school and college athletes, Med Sci Sports Exerc 1995: 25: 641-7

Weidenbener, EJ, Krauss, MD, Waller, BF et al, Incorporation of screening echocardiography in the preparticipation exam, Clin J Sports Med 1995;5 (2): 86-89

Wiggins, DL, Wiggins, ME, The Female Athlete, Clin Sports Med 1997; 16: 593-612

Rehabilitation:

Functional Anatomy of the Limbs and back, 6th edition, David B. Jenkins, PhD, Department of Biomedical Sciences, Section of Anatomy, Southern Illinois University 1991

Physical Medicine and Rehabilitation, NYU School of Medicine and Rusk Institute of Rehabilitation Medicine, March 2000

Women:

ACSM Position Stand on the Female Athlete Triad, Med. Sci. Sports Exerc, Vol29 (5): I – ix 1997

American College of Obstetrics and Gynecology, Guidelines for Exercise during pregnancy and the postpartum period: ACOG technical bulletin 189. Washington DC, ACOG 1994

American Pyschiatric Association, Diagnostic & Statistical Manual of Mental Disorders, 4th edition, American Psychiatric Asociation, Washington, D.C. 1994

DeCree, C, Steroid Metabolism and Menstrual Irregularities in the Exercising Female: A Review, Sports Medicine 1998 Jun 25 (6): 369 -406

Joy, E, Clark, N, Ireland, ML, Martire, J et al, Team Management of the Female Athlete Triad, Part II: Optimal Treatment and Prevention Tactics, The Physician and Sportsmedicine, April 1997; Vol 25 (4): 55-69

Schultz, V, Hansel, R, Tyler, VE, Rational Phytotherapy: A Physician's Guide to Herbal Medicine, 3rd edition, Springer-Verlag 1998

Smith, A.D., The Female Athlete Triad: Causes, Diagnosis and Treatment, The Physician and Sportsmedicine, July 1996; Vol 24 (7): 67-86

Speroff, L, Glass RH, Kase NG, In: Mitchell, C (ed) Amenorrhea, Clinical Gynecologic Endocrinology & Infertility, Sixth edition, Lippincott, Williams and Wilkins, Baltimore, Md 1999: 421-485

Wiggins, DL, Wiggins ME, The Female Athlete, In: Clinics in Sports Medicine: Primary Care of the Injured Athlete, Pt II Vol 16 (4): 1997 pgs 593 -601

Special Athletes:

ABLEDATA Database od Assistive Technology. Winter Sports & recreational Equipment Fact Sheet #16. National Institute on Disability & Rehabilitation Research 1993

American Academy of Pediatrics Committee on Sports Medicine and Fitness. Atlantoaxial Instability in Down Syndrome: Subject Review, Pediatrics 1995: 96 (1) 151 – 154

American Academy of Pediatrics Committee on Children with Disabilities. General Principles in the Care of Children and Adolescents with Genetic Disorder and Other Chronic Health Conditions, Pediatrics, 1997; 99: 4, 643 -644

American Academy of Pediatrics Committee on Sports Medicine and Fitness. Sports Medicine: Health Care for Young Athletes – 2nd edition, Elk Grove Village, Il, American Academy of Pediatrics 1991

Broadrick, T, Play Ball ! Exceptional Parent, 1997; 27 (7), 40 – 43

Broadrick,T, Hockey Time is Here, Exceptional Parent 1998; 28 (12), 54-55

Burkor, C.K., We Want to Play Too ! Including All Children in Youth Sports and Complying with the ADA, Exceptional Parent 1998; 28:6, 72 -75

Carter, GT, Rehabilitation Management in Neuromuscular Disease, Journal Neurological Rehabilitation 1997; 11: 69-80

Chamilian, D., Gooaaaaal! Ball. Exceptional Parent 2000: 30 (8) 32 -33

Chamilian, D., Tee Time for All, Exceptional Parent 2000; 30 (5), 74 -77

Chamalian, D., "Top" of their Game, Exceptional Parent, 2000: 30;(9): 90-92

Colon, KM, Sports and Recreation: Many Rewards, but barriers exist, Exceptional Parent. 1998; 28(3): 56-60

Duncan,CC, Ogle, EM, Spina Bifida In: Goldberg, B, ed, Sports and Exercise for Children with Chronic Health Conditions, Champaign, Il: Human Kinetics 1995; 79 -88

Dykens EM, Cohen DJ, Effects of Special Olympics International on Social Competance in Persons with Mental Retardation, Journal American Academy of Child & Adolescent Psychiatry 1996: 35: 223-229

Empire State Games for the Physically Challenged. Long Island Regional Competition. NYS Office of Parks, Recreation and Historic Preservation 1998

Exceptional Parent Fitness Column. Motor Sports Activities & Sports Skills: Age Appropriate, Functional & Fun, Exceptional Parent, 1990; 20 (3) 50 – 52

Goldberg, MJ, Participating in Special Olympics. American Academy of Orthopedic Surgeons Bulletin 1995, 43 :3

Hack, C.H., Paradigms of Care for Children with Special Healthcare Needs, Pediatric Annals, 1997; 26: 11, 674 -8

Kilmer, DD, McDonald, CM, Childhood Progressive Neuromuscular Disease, In: Goldberg, B, Sports and Exercise for Children with Chronic Health Conditions, Champaign, Il: Human Kinetics 1995; 109 – 121

Lamphear, NE, Liptak, GS, Weitzman, M, Impact of Chronic Health Conditions in Childhood, In: Goldberg, B. ed, Sports and Exercise for Children with Chronic Health Cobditions. Champaign, Il: Human Kinetics 1995; 3-12

Liptak, G.S., Revell, G.M. Community Physican's Role in Case Management of Children with Chronic Illnesses, Pediatrics 1989; 84:3, 465 -471

Little, J, Gaebler-Spira, D, Cerebral Palsy & Sports, Exceptional Parent 1996: 26 (8) 53 - 55

Mayo, R, Easy Riders, Exceptional Parent, 2000; 30 (4) 55 -57

Mushett, CA, Wyeth, DO, Richter, KJ, Cerebral Palsy In: Goldberg, B ed, Sports and Exercise for Children with Chronic Health Conditions, Champaign, Il: Human Kinetics 1995; 123 -134

Nelson, MA, Harris, SS, The Benefits and Risks of Sports and Exercise for Children with Chronic Health Conditions, In: Goldberg, B., ed. Sports and Exercise for Children with Chronic Health Conditions, Champaign, IL: Human Kinetics 1995; 13-30

Palfrey, J, Haynie, M, Managed Care and Children with Special Health Care Needs: Creating a Medical Home. American Academy of Pediatrics 1998

Perrin, J.M., Chronic Illness, In: Levine, M.D., Carey, W.B., Crocker, A.C., ed, Developmental – Behavioral Pediatrics 2nd ed., Philadelphia: W.B. Saunders Co. 1992; 304 – 308

Peuschel, SM The Child with Down Syndrome, In: Levine MD, Carey, WB, Crocker, AC eds, Developmental Behavioral Pediatrics, 2nd edition Philadelphia: WB Saunders 1992; 221 -228

Pianoforte, K, Horsin Around, Exceptional Parent 2000; 30 (11): 80- 83

Pimentel, A.E., The Family System in Developmental Disabilities In: Capute, AJ, Accardo PJ eds, Developmental Disabilities in Infancy & Childhood, Baltimore: Paul H Brookes 1991: 189 – 196

Privett, C, The Special Olympics: A Tradition of Excellence. Exceptional Parent 1999; 29:5, 28-36

Shea, A, A Moving Experience, Exceptional Parent 1998; 28 (5) 53 -55

Stoling, J, The Challenge to be Great, Exceptional Parent 1998; 28 (5) 42-45

Taft, L.T., Matthew, W.S., Cerebral Palsy, In: Levine M.D., Carey, W.B., Crocker, A.C., eds, Developmental – Behavioral Pediatrics, 2nd edition, Philadelphia, WB Saunders 1992; 527 -534

Geriatrics

Christmas, C, Andersen, Exercise and older patients: Guidelines for the Clinician, J Am Geriatr. Soc 48: 318-324, 2000

Kendall/ Hunt, Geriatrics R Syllabus 4th edition, American Geriatric Society, Iowa 1999

Sutton, JR, Brock, RM (eds), Sports Medicine for the Mature Athlete, Benchmark Press, Indiana 1986

Infectious Disease Issues

Feigin RD, Cherry JC,(ed), Textbook of Pediatric Infectious Diseases 4th edition, WB Saunders, Phil, PA, 1998

Pickering, LK(ed), 2000 Red Book: report of the Committee on Infectious Diseases 25th edition, American Academy of Pediatrics, Elk grove, Il 2000

Sports Psychology

American Psychiatric Association: DSM-IV Washington, DC 1993

Anshel, M, Sport Psychology; From theory to practice, Gorsuch Scarisbrick, Scottsdale, Ariz 1990

Eccles, JS, Sex differences in achievement patterns. IN: Sonderegger, T (ed) Nebraska symposium on motivation 1984: Psychology and Gender. Lincoln University of Nebraska Press 1984

Horn, T (ed), Advances in Sport Psychology, Champaign, Ill, Human Kinetics 1992

Jackson, S, Athletes in flow: A qualitative investigation of flow states in elite figure skaters. Journal of Applied Sport Psychology; 7:333-345, 1992

Johnson, MD, Disordered eating in active and athletic women, Clinics in Sports Medicine 13 (2) 355-369 1994

Larson, GA, Starkey, C, Zaichkowsky, LD, Psychological Aspects of Athletic Injuries perceived by athletic trainers, The Sports Psychologist 10; 37-47 1996

McGrath, JE, Social and Psychological Factors in Stress, Holt, Rinehart & Winston, NY, NY 1970

Nadeau, CH, Halliwell, WR, Newell, KM, Roberts, GC (ed) Psychology of Motor Development and Sport, Human Kinetics, Champaign, Ill 1980

Nideffer, RM, The Inner Athlete, Crowell, NY, NY 1976

Rushall, BS, Psyching in Sports, Pelham, London 1979

Weinberg RS, Gould, D, Sports and Exercise Psychology, Champaign, Ill, Human Kinetics 1995

Yukelson, D, Weinberg, Jackson, A, A multidimensional group cohesion instrument for intercollegiate basketball teams, J Sports Psychology 6: 103 -117, 1984

Environmental Illnesses

Auerbach, PS, Wilderness Medicine, Management of Wilderness and Environmental Emergencies, 3rd edition, Mosby Publishers 1995

Forgey, William, Wilderness Medicine, 4th edition, Beyond First Aid, ICS Books Inc, Merrillville, Indiana 1994

Forgey, William (ed) , Wilderness Medical Society Practice Guidelines, 2nd edition, Globe Pequot Press, Guilford, Connecticut 2000

Tintinalli, J, Rothstein, R, Krome, R, (ed), Emergency Medicine, McGraw-Hill Books, 1985

Rivers, C, Weber, D, Kreplick, L, (ed), Preparing for the Written Board Exam in Emergency Medicine, 2nd edition, Emergency Medicine Educational Enterprises, Inc, Milford, Ohio 1997

Cardiopulmonary Resuscitation

Advanced trauma Life Support, 6th edition, American College of Surgeons, Chicago, Il 1997

Chamiedes, L, Hazinki, MF, Pediatric Advanced Life Support 1997-1999, American Heart Association, Dallas 1997

Cummins, R, Advanced Cardiac Life Support 1997 -1999, American Heart Association, Dallas 1997

Jun, Kathleen (ed), Currents in Emergency Cardiovascular Care, Guidelines 2000 for Cardiopulmonary Resuscitation & Emergency Cardiovascular Care, Volume 11, no. 3, Fall 2000

Scuderi, G, McCann, P, Bruno, P, Sports Medicine: Principles of Primary Care, Mosby, NY 1997

Exercise Testing

McArdle, W.D., Katch, F.I., Katch, V..L., Exercise Physiology, Energy, Nutrition and Human Performance, Lea and Febiger, Philadelphia 1991

Wasserman,K, Hansen, J.E., Sue, D.Y., Whipp, B.J., Casaburi, R, Principles of Exercise Testing and Interpretation, Lea and Fibiger, Philadelphia, 1994

Roca, J, Whipp, B.J., Clinical Exercise Testing, European Respiratory Monograph, Volume 2, Monograph 6, 1997 (1 -164)

Casting & Splinting

Miller, A, Petrizzi, MJ, Petrizzi, MG, " Three Way " splint for acute ankle injury, Phys Sports Med 2000; 28(6): 99-100

Rockwood, Jr, , C A, Green, DP, (ed) Fractures in Adults, 2nd edition, Vol, I, II, III

Petrizzi, MJ, Petrizzi, MG, Making a Tension Night Splint for Plantar Fasciitis, Phys and Sports Med 1998; 26(6): 113-114

Petrizzi, MJ, Petrizzi, MG, Making an Ulnar Gutter Splint for a Boxer's Fracture, Phys and Spots Med 1999; 27(1): 111 -112

Petrizzi, MJ, Shahady, E, (ed) , Sports Medicine for Coaches and Trainers, 1st edition

Injections & aspirations

Anderson, Bruce, Kaye, S, Treatment of Flexor Tenosynovitis of the Hand with Corticosteroids, Archives of Internal Medicine, 1991: 151 – 156

Anderson, L, Aspirating and Injecting the Acutely Painful Joint, Emergency Medicine, Jan 15, 1991

Gilbert, D, Moellering, R, Snade, M, Sanford Guide to Antimicrobial Therapy, 31st edition, 2001: 22-23

Owen, DS, Weiss, JJ, Wilke, WS, When to Aspirate and Inject Joints, Patient Care, Sept. 1990

Pfenninger, J, A Review of Joint Aspiration and Injection, AAFP 1991 Scientific Assembly

Protective and Supportive Equipment

Benson, M, (ed) , Protective Equipment, In: 1997-1998 NCAA Sports Medicine handbook.Overland Park, KS: The National Collegiate Athletic Association, 1997

Berg, R, Berkey DB, Tang JM et al, Knowledge and attitudes of Arizona high school coaches regarding oral – facial injuries and mouthguard use among athletes, J Am Dent Assoc 1998 Oct;129(10): 1425-32

Cheng, TL, Fields, CB, Brenner, RA et al, Sports Injuries: An important cause of morbidity in urban youth, Pediatrics 2000 Mar; 105(3): E32

Gross, MT et al, Effect of ankle orthoses on functional performance for individuals with recurrent lateral ankle sprains, JOSPT 1997; 25(4): 245-252

In Line Skating injuries in children and adolescents. AAP Committee on Injury and Poison Prevention and Committee on Sports Medicine and Fitness, Pediatrics 1998 Apr; 101:720-2

Knorr, HL, Jonas, JB, Retinal detachments by squash ball accidents, Am J Ophthalmol 1996 Aug; 122(2): 260-1

Livingston, LA, Forbes, SL, Eye Injuries in Women's lacrosse: strict rule reinforcement and mandatory eyewear required, J Trauma 1996 Jan; 40(1): 144-5

Machold, W, Kwasny, O, Gassler, P et al, Risk of injury through snowboarding, J Trauma, 2000 Jun;48(6): 1109-14

Orenstein, JB, Injuries and small wheel skates, Ann Emerg Med 1996 Feb; 27 (2): 204-209

Rice, MR, Alvanos, l, Kenney, B, Snowmobile injuries and deaths in children: a review of national injury data and state legislation, Pediatrics 2000 Mar; 105: 615-619

Saliba, E, Foreman, S, Abadie, RT, Jr, Protective equipment consideration, In: Athletic Injuries and rehabilitation, WB Saunders 1996

Schrieber, RA, Branche – Dorsey CM, Ryan, GW et al, Risk Factors for injuries from in-line skating and the effectiveness of safety gear, NEJM 1996 Nov 28;335(22): 1630-5

Shafi, F, Gilbert, JC, Loghmanee, F et al, Impact of bicycle safety helmet legislation on children admitted to a regional pediatric trauma center, J Pediatr Surg 1998 Feb;33(2): 317-21

Thompson, DC, Nunn, ME, Thompson, RS, Rivara, FP, Effectiveness of bicycle safety helmets in preventing serious facial injury, JAMA 1996 Dec 25: 276(24): 1974-5

Thompson, MJ, Rivara, FP, Bicycle related injuries, Am Fam Physician, 2001, May 15; 63(10): 2007-2014

Wichman, S, Martin, DRE, Bracing for Activity, Phys Sportsmed 1996; 24(9): 88-94